# FAST FACTS FOR
# THE RADIOLOGY NURSE

**Valerie Aarne Grossman, MALS, BSN, RN,** is a registered nurse with more than 3 decades of diverse nursing experience including direct patient care, hospital leadership, professional service, and writing for publication. She has worked in a variety of settings, from the emergency department to intensive care to radiology. She has volunteered her services to such valued groups as the Emergency Nurses Association, the Association for Radiologic & Imaging Nursing, RAD-AID.org, and the National Certification Corporation, as well as serving on such boards as the Research Subject Review Board at the University of Rochester and the New York State Board of Nursing. She is the author of numerous peer-reviewed articles, chapters, books, and online pieces, and is a manuscript reviewer for a number of international publishers. Her passion for direct patient caregivers drives her involvement in projects that improve the tools and information made available for colleagues taking care of patients. She believes that health care providers (especially nurses) are "scientists who touch patients" as well as "scientists who *are touched by* patients," and works to provide the intellectual information that feeds their professional curiosity.

# FAST FACTS FOR THE RADIOLOGY NURSE

## An Orientation and Nursing Care Guide in a Nutshell

Valerie Aarne Grossman, MALS, BSN, RN

Editor

**SPRINGER PUBLISHING COMPANY**

Springer Publishing Company, LLC
11 West 42nd Street
New York, NY 10036
www.springerpub.com

*Acquisitions Editor*: Elizabeth Nieginski
*Composition*: S4Carlisle Publishing Services

ISBN: 978-0-8261-2936-9
*e-book ISBN*: 978-0-8261-2937-6

14 15 16 / 5 4 3 2 1

The author and the publisher of this Work have made every effort to use sources believed to be reliable to provide information that is accurate and compatible with the standards generally accepted at the time of publication. Because medical science is continually advancing, our knowledge base continues to expand. Therefore, as new information becomes available, changes in procedures become necessary. We recommend that the reader always consult current research and specific institutional policies before performing any clinical procedure. The author and publisher shall not be liable for any special, consequential, or exemplary damages resulting, in whole or in part, from the readers' use of, or reliance on, the information contained in this book. The publisher has no responsibility for the persistence or accuracy of URLs for external or third-party Internet websites referred to in this publication and does not guarantee that any content on such websites is, or will remain, accurate or appropriate.

**Library of Congress Cataloging-in-Publication Data**

Fast facts for the radiology nurse : an orientation and nursing care guide in a nutshell / [edited by] Valerie Aarne Grossman.
    p. ; cm. — (Fast facts)
Includes bibliographical references and index.
ISBN-13: 978-0-8261-2936-9
ISBN-10: 0-8261-2936-6
ISBN-13: 978-0-8261-2937-6 (e-book)
    I. Grossman, Valerie G. A., editor of compilation. II. Series: Fast facts (Springer Publishing Company)
    [DNLM: 1. Radiology. 2. Specialties, Nursing. 3. Nursing Care—methods.   WY 150]
RC78.7.D53
616.07'57—dc23
                    2014004342

Printed in the United States of America by Gasch Printing.

*This book is dedicated to the countless individuals who bestowed on me the privilege of being their nurse. From Jackie, Anne, and Mrs. S. in the early (and most imprintable) years of my nursing career, to journeys that are more recent with Meghan, Shea, Gail, and "Tallahassee ZZ": You shared your innermost views of the world with me, you trusted your lives to my scientific abilities, you looked at life's finality with me next to you . . . you changed me . . . I can only hope that I have in some way helped you.*

*I also dedicate this book to my parents (Marie and John Aarne) and my daughters (Sarah and Nicole Grossman): You give my days purpose and add color to my life's rainbow. Thank you for making a difference.*

# Contents

## Part III: Radiologic Imaging Modalities: CT and MRI

## Part IV: Interventional Radiology

## Part V: Diagnostic and Other Imaging Modalities

## Part VI: Special Issues in Radiology Nursing

## Part VII: Emerging Areas of Radiology Nursing

# Contributors

**John P. Deveikis, MD, PA**
Professor
Department of Neurosurgery
Department of Radiology
University of Alabama
Birmingham, Alabama

**Susan Deveikis, RN, BSN**
Clinical Care Coordinator
Department of Neurosurgery
University of Alabama
Birmingham, Alabama

**Brooke Grandusky-Green, RN, BSN**
Analyst/Programmer
Department of Imaging Sciences
University of Rochester Medical Center
Rochester, New York

**Mohammed Mohsin Khadir, MD**
Department of Imaging Sciences
University of Rochester Medical Center (URMC)
Rochester, New York

**Andrew Mangiacapre, RN, BSN**
Staff Nurse
Interventional Radiology
Highland Hospital (URMC affiliate)
Staff Nurse
Interventional Radiology
University Imaging at Science Park (URMC affiliate)
Rochester, New York

**Anna C. Montejano, RN, MSNEd, CEN**
Faculty
Sutter Center for Health Professions
Sacramento, California
Educator
TriageFirst
Fairview, North Carolina

**Lora K. Ott, PhD, RN**
Assistant Professor
Indiana University of Pennsylvania
Indiana, Pennsylvania

**Ayman Sawas, MD**
Department of Imaging Sciences
University of Rochester Medical Center
Rochester, New York

**Ashwani Kumar Sharma, MD, MBBS**
Assistant Professor
Interventional Radiology
University of Rochester Medical Center
Rochester, New York

**Labib H. Syed, MD, MPH**
Assistant Professor
Interventional Radiology
University of Rochester Medical Center
Rochester, New York

**Lynn Sayre Visser, MSN, RN, CEN, CPEN**
Staff Nurse
Sutter Roseville Medical Center
Roseville, California
Staff Nurse
Sutter Medical Center
Sacramento, California
Educator
TriageFirst
Fairview, North Carolina

**Polly Gerber Zimmermann, RN, MS, MBA, CEN, FAEN**
Associate Professor
Harry S Truman College
Chicago, Illinois

# Reviewers

**Meredith J. Addison, RN, MSN, CEN, FAEN**
Staff Nurse
Emergency Department
Regional Hospital
Terre Haute, Indiana

**Melissa Brongo, RN, AAS**
Staff Nurse
Medical Imaging
Highland Hospital (URMC affiliate)
Rochester, New York

**Yvette Conyers, RN, MS, FNP-C, CTN-B**
Clinical Instructor
University of Rochester Medical Center School of Nursing
Rochester, New York

**Sarah L. Grossman, BS**
Senior Direct Support Professional
Heritage Christian Services
Rochester, New York

**Jena N. Hlad, RN, BSN, BA, MBA**
Staff Nurse
Critical Care
Aureus Medical Staffing
Omaha, Nebraska

**John Loughner, PharmD**
University of Rochester Medical Center
Rochester, New York

**Velecia Marston, RN, AAS**
Staff Nurse
Medical Imaging
Highland Hospital (affiliate of the University of Rochester)
Rochester, New York

**Mark R. O'Connell, RN, BS, PCCN**
Staff Nurse
Emergency Department
Newark-Wayne Community Hospital
Newark, New York

**Lynn Sayre Visser, MSN, BS, CEN, CPEN, CLNC**
Staff Nurse
Sutter Roseville Medical Center
Roseville, California
Staff Nurse
Sutter Medical Center
Sacramento, California
Educator
TriageFirst
Fairview, North Carolina

**Joann Zicari, RN, BSN**
Staff Nurse
Medical Imaging
Highland Hospital
Rochester, New York
Circulator Nurse
Private practice, John D. Ritrosky, MD
Fort Myers, Florida

# Foreword

An increasing number of nurses work in radiology departments or other imaging areas, and this innovative handbook provides a concise yet comprehensive resource addressing the many roles the nurse fills within the imaging areas. This handbook will also serve as an important primer for nurses who are novices in radiology and imaging areas and as a valuable reference for nurses with radiology experience.

An experienced radiology nurse clinician, nurse manager, and published author, Ms. Grossman, editor of *Fast Facts for the Radiology Nurse,* has a passion for nursing and an inexhaustible commitment to elevate her chosen professional specialty of radiology nursing. Ms. Grossman has put together a concise handbook that covers the most basic concepts in radiology nursing and provides information on specific procedures.

This book covers many topics essential to the success of the nurse working in an imaging setting. Radiology nurses are vital to the success of the department's team, and every radiology nurse needs knowledge of radiation's ability to show diagnostic information and uses in treatment, but also have an awareness of its potential for harm that necessitates vigilance for safety.

The book offers information regarding the basic skills that a radiology nurse uses in everyday practice. Nurses draw from prior critical care and/or emergency nursing knowledge and assessment skills in radiology, and also learn new skills specific to the imaging environment including vascular access, hemostasis, infection control, physiological monitoring, and documentation. Important information on sedation and analgesia includes medications in easy-to-read tables. Complete sections on caring for patients who are having computed tomography or magnetic resonance imaging scans as well as interventional radiology procedures are covered with essential information for the reader. Other areas of radiology are also discussed.

"Fast Facts in a Nutshell" boxes, located throughout the book, highlight information that is essential to know. In summary, this handbook is a welcome addition to the resources for radiology nursing, which are few in number compared to other specialties. The handbook's size makes it easily portable as a bedside reference. A copy of this handbook would be an important addition to any radiology nursing unit's resources and would be useful in emergency and critical care unit libraries as well.

*Kathleen A. Gross, MSN, RN-BC, CRN*
*Editor,* Journal of Radiology Nursing

# Preface

Many nurses who enter the imaging arena come from vastly different backgrounds in the profession. I have worked with mental health nurses, pediatric nurses, critical care nurses, and emergency care nurses who have transitioned into radiology nurses. They all bring unique experience to our departments; all have great value. Individually it may be tough; yet being part of a diverse nursing team makes us strong and determined to provide the very best in patient care. As you know, radiology is a great place to work. A bad day in radiology is often better than the best day on the floors. It just is.

Learning to be a radiology nurse takes us out of our "comfort zone" and immerses us in a world developed by physicians and technologists. It's all about getting great images so that radiologists can make perfect diagnoses for the patients we serve. Yet, when nurses are introduced to the environment, some teams struggle with the diversity of practice styles and goals. The *Journal of Radiology Nursing* diligently works to provide nurses with up-to-date information regarding our focus of practice. The core curriculum has been developed from the knowledge of a vast nursing team. We utilize information from the American College of Radiology, the Society of Interventional Radiology, and many other organizations to enhance our knowledge. What we as radiology nurses haven't had until now is a book—a book that we can put in our pocket and use to teach newer nurses or one that provides a quick-glance resource for the more seasoned nurse.

*Fast Facts for the Radiology Nurse* was written to serve the needs of nurses in a variety of imaging settings. Basic information such as vascular access, infection control, teamwork, and sterile technique is covered. Caring for patients from the emergency department or intensive care unit poses different types of challenges for the radiology nurse, and this book offers ways to provide care safely to these patients as well. Every patient can present a particular challenge in radiology, so there are tips for caring for young patients, older patients, large patients, emotionally stressed patients . . . ideas for nearly all situations.

Much of what we do in radiology centers around computed tomography, magnetic resonance imaging, and interventional radiology (IR) and, therefore, this book focuses heavily on those areas—from safety around contrast, magnets, and radiation to particular information on over 50 different IR procedures we perform for our patients. Contributors with clinical expertise from a variety of settings have assisted with this book, creating a well-researched, reviewed, and polished text for the reader. This book presents all the facts that the radiology nurse needs to be able to jump feet first into the clinical setting.

*Valerie Aarne Grossman*

# Acknowledgments

This book could not have happened if it were not for the passion, perseverance, and belief in the "frontline nurse" that my editor, Elizabeth Nieginski, possesses. There are not enough words in this language to describe her constant support and belief in this project. She granted me the right to enjoy this project, to roll with the punches, to jump those hurdles, and to be proud of what we are giving to our readers.

Following Elizabeth's excellent leadership was my team of contributors and reviewers. Your passion for excellent care at the bedside translated so nicely into the words contained here. Your critical eyes for what the nursing reader would need to know to provide care to the radiology patient behind every image were precise in every possible manner. It takes a team with high moral standards that believes in the very best of patient care to walk with our patients through their journeys in health, injury, and sickness: You all make a difference for our patients. Thank you for believing in this project!

To my favorite librarians who make every literature search a successful and bountiful one! Bonnie Archer and Lorraine Procello: Your belief in the bedside nurse makes us better at what we do, what we learn, and what we can provide to every patient we serve.

To my writing mentors over the years: Without you, this book wouldn't exist. Donna Ojanen Thomas, Dr. Frank Edwards, Polly Gerber Zimmermann, Gail Lenehan, Julie Briggs, and Susan Hollis . . . thank you for walking me to the doors of opportunity, and teaching me how to cross those difficult thresholds.

# I

# Radiology Foundation

# 1

# Introduction to Radiology Nursing and Safety

## Valerie Aarne Grossman

In this chapter, you will discover:

1. The complexity of radiology nursing
2. The essential role of teamwork
3. Safe radiation practices

The world of radiology is changing very quickly. It wasn't too long ago when the only caregivers in any given radiology department were the radiologist and the technologist. Now, however, there may be a complex team of transporters, unlicensed assistive personnel, nurses, technologists, midlevel providers (nurse practitioners and physician assistants), as well as the radiologists! As the complexity of health care grows, so too does imaging ability. Different modalities, different technologies, and different skill levels must all work in harmony to provide precision images for the radiologist, who will ultimately provide insight into a patient's condition for the ordering physician. Decreasing reimbursement, increasing regulation, and increasing sophistication combined with the different practice styles and needs of the radiology modalities can lead to a very confusing nursing environment that is continually changing and ever challenging (Donnelly, Dickerson, Goodfriend, & Muething, 2010).

Nursing is quickly gaining a greater presence in radiology settings. The increasing complexity of procedures within the modalities, as well as patients with more complex health care issues, requires the expertise of motivated nursing professionals. Radiology nurses must be self-motivated, patient focused, and able to work with a diverse team of individuals. Often, nurses in radiology are breaking new ground, discovering new patient care issues, and amending practice to meet new regulations. A radiology nurse must be able to care for the widest range of patients (much like a nurse in the emergency department), from pediatric to geriatric, from trauma to oncology, from self-care to total-care patients . . . there is no routine in radiology. Yet, it is more than that. A radiology nurse must remember that there is a person behind each and every image . . . someone with a life that matters, a story worth sharing. In the chaos of a normal work day, it can sometimes be easy for the nurse to forget how the patient sees his or her visit to radiology: *Will this scan show that there is a tumor? Will this ultrasound show that I'm pregnant? Can this interventional radiology procedure stop the bleeding?* Our radiology environment is "normal" for us, but to our patients who trust us with their lives it is foreign and scary. It is our role as professionals to guide patients through their time with us in radiology and to treat them with dignity and respect.

## *FAST FACTS in a NUTSHELL*

Refrain from the use of personal electronic devices while in the clinical area. This is an infection control risk and may allow the patients/visitors to misperceive where your attention is focused.

## RADIATION SAFETY

Today's advancing medical imaging arenas are providing physicians with state-of-the-art technology to see within a body through diagnostic imaging tools. Yet, with that ability comes a degree of risk. It falls to the radiology team to protect not only the patient but also themselves in this environment. Some simple rules should be followed 100% of the time when working with radiation in the areas of computed tomography (CT), positron emission tomography (PET), interventional radiology, x-ray, nuclear medicine, mammography, cardiac catheter lab, operating room with a C-arm, or any number of other settings.

The very common term "ALARA" (as low as reasonably achievable) refers to the recommendation that the technologist uses the lowest amount of radiation technique possible to achieve the image that the radiologist needs. This is not a "one-step" process, as there are times when it may involve utilizing other modalities that do not use radiation (ultrasound or magnetic resonance imaging [MRI]). If the best study for the patient is one that uses radiation, then the team must consider increasing the distance from the source of radiation, decreasing the time of exposure to radiation, and using the appropriate shielding of the patient or staff.

- **Time**:
  - Decreasing the amount of exposure time will automatically decrease the dose of radiation to the patient and the provider.
  - Thorough planning of the image or the procedure will be necessary, with streamlined work flow, precise protocols, and operational expertise of the equipment and/or radioactive material by the technologist.

- **Distance**:
  - Increasing the distance from the source of radiation will decrease the exposure dose.

- **Shielding**:
  - Using the appropriate type of shielding will protect the individual from exposure. There are a variety of products available, including lead aprons, lead shielding stands, goggles, thyroid shields, and sterile drapes that cover the patients during procedures (Association of periOperative Registered Nurses, Conner, & Blanchard, 2011).

*FAST FACTS in a NUTSHELL*

With mounting concerns of the carcinogenic effects of imaging techniques, it is essential for all imaging providers to keep as a priority the safety of staff and patients through utilization of the lowest dose possible for the imaging outcome desired, as well as ALARA.

# 2

# Essentials of Teamwork

## Polly Gerber Zimmermann

In this chapter, you will discover:

1. How to promote "team"
2. How to set boundaries with coworkers
3. How to handle escalating behavior

## TEAMWORK

"There is no 'I' in team" is a common but often impotent phrase. To create a group that wants the same goals there must be an atmosphere that promotes comfort, camaraderie, and security with coworkers who are comfortable speaking up while supporting patient safety and quality care.

## BUILDING TEAMWORK

- Communicate reasons to enhance pride and tradition in the department.

- People don't worry about being fired as much as falling into disfavor or not belonging to the group.
- Compliment in public; criticize in private.
  - Identify at least one thing for each department member that the person does well and mention it in front of others.
- Look for an opportunity to tell other people's bosses how well they did: It *will* get back to them.
- Find something outside of work that is important to each person in the department.
  - Regularly discuss that topic with them so your only interaction isn't work. Common subjects include children/grandchildren, hobbies, or vacation.
- Consider a department meeting where universal expectations and code of conduct are identified, agreed upon, and posted.
  - Hold everyone accountable.

## DEALING WITH CHANGE: THE ONE CONSTANT IN LIFE IS CHANGE

- Involve the affected individuals when determining change.
- Appeal to higher core, common values, such as "safe patient care," "quality," or "effectiveness." Who would ever publicly admit they don't care about those motivators?
- Communicate the reason for the change.
- Work privately to build a supportive consensus before any public presentation.
  - Start with the early adopters.
- Know best practices and cite them, as it shows what is possible.
- Cite a higher authority when asking for change or agreement. Sources can include:
  - Professional association recommendations
  - A published article
  - A senior administrator
  - What other hospitals in the local area are doing
  - Regulations
  - Lawsuits

"Bullying" or "disruptive behavior" is no longer acceptable in health care either by staff or patients/families. It is not only demoralizing but affects the quality of care. In one study, 76% of respondents reported that disruptive behaviors were linked to adverse events such as medical errors (71%) and patient mortality (27%) (Roche, Diers, Duffield, & Catling-Paull, 2010).

## FAST FACTS in a NUTSHELL

- Say something positive as the first thing you say to everyone every day.
- Establish behavioral policies and expectations, such as chain of command and/or zero-tolerance.
- Focus on improving the process rather than the person.

# DEALING WITH "DISRUPTIVE" HEALTH CARE PROVIDERS

## Verbal and Nonverbal Abuse

### Signs

- Sighing, rolling eyes
- Abrupt response/walking away while another professional is talking
- Sarcasm, snide remarks
- Talking behind someone's back
- Undermining/withholding information

### Responsive Behaviors

- Deal with the action and request what you expect. Practice these phrases to use, especially if new to the department.
    - "I sense that there may be something you wanted to say to me. It's okay to speak directly to me."
    - "The individuals I learn the most from are clearer in their directions and feedback. Is there some way we can structure this type of situation?"
    - "When something happens that is 'different' or 'contrary' to what I thought or understood it leaves me with questions. Help me understand how this situation may have happened."

- "It is my understanding that there was more information available regarding this situation. I believe if I had known that, it would affect how I learn."
- Use assertive communication with "I" statements that address behaviors (not personality).
  - "I've noticed ____."
  - "When you do____, I feel ____."
  - "I need you to ____."
- Use TeamSTEPPS's Advocacy and Assertion (http://team stepps.ahrg.gov). It outlines the steps to take. when you are *C*oncerned, *U*ncomfortable, or recognize a *S*afety concern (*CUS*) about what is currently happening.
  - Make an opening.
  - State the concern.
  - Offer a corrective action in a firm and respectful manner.
  - Obtain an agreement.
  - If ignored, *repeat the request a second time.* If not satisfied, then take stronger action such as activating the chain of command.

## FAST FACTS in a NUTSHELL

Up to 80% of the time, nurses deal with difficulties by avoidance. Besides the stress of unresolved conflict, failing to address inappropriate behaviors creates a culture where deviancy is "normalized."

## Specific-Person Abuse

### Signs

- Specific negative language or behavior directed toward an individual, including sexual harassment.
- Screaming, throwing things, profanity.

### Responsive Behaviors

- Tell the person to stop.
- Tell the person the discussion must be had in private. Turn around and walk away.
- "Code White/Code Pink," where all staff members surround a verbally attacked staff member. They stand silent with arms

crossed and stare at the disruptive individual, who usually stops the offending behavior.

═══════════════════════════════════*FAST FACTS in a NUTSHELL*

An ounce of prevention is worth a pound of cure when dealing with upset patients or family members. Set the positive tone from the first contact.

## PATIENT/FAMILY GENERAL HINTS

- Look up and beam when greeting people (keep the area over your heart open).
- Consider a scripted apology ("I'm sorry you had to wait") anytime you do not immediately take the patient in.
- Compliment parents on their children. (All parents think their children are good looking and above average!)
- Remark to a child about "how big" they are.
- Do not interrupt the person when he or she is speaking to you.
  - The average health care provider interrupts 23 seconds into the patient's statement.

## DEALING WITH "DISRUPTIVE PATIENTS/FAMILIES"

Disruptive behavior is on a continuum. Recognize escalation and intervene appropriately.

### First Stage: Challenging the Provider

#### Signs

- Voice changes tone, volume, or cadence from normal conversation.
- Body language demonstrates muscle tenseness, anger expression, or leaning forward.

#### De-escalation Responses

- Ignore challenges to the nurse's qualifications or actions; redirect to the issue at hand to avoid a power struggle.

- Do not quote authoritative rules.
  - "You can't act like that! This is a hospital," rarely changes behavior.
- Let the person vent and do not deny the complaint to "deflate" the emotion.
- Acknowledge the person's emotions ("I can see you are angry") so the person feels validated.
- Use the person's name often, as it grabs the rational part of the brain.
- Consider a "blameless apology"—"I am sorry you had a problem." Seek to move forward, "What can we do now to get you the care you need?"

## Second Stage: Refusal and Noncompliance

### Signs

- Becomes more argumentative and challenging.

### De-escalation Responses

- Set limits and specifically name unacceptable behavior (threatening, swearing). "I felt put down by your sarcastic comment about _____. I treat you in a respectful manner and I need you to do the same when you interact with me."
- Consider a verbal contract to control behavior. ("Can you do _____ while I do _____?")
- Focus on concrete needs (cup of coffee, and so on).

## Third Stage: Emotional Release

### Signs

- Outburst, with higher intensity.
- Loss of rational thought.

### De-escalation Responses

- Remove from public arena.
- Restate what the person is saying.

- Share your emotional response ("Now you are scaring me"). It may make the person realize, perhaps for the first time, that he or she is losing control.
- Give undivided attention.

## Fourth Stage: Intimidation

### Signs

- Verbal or nonverbal threats.
- You feel frightened in your gut: trust your gut.

### De-escalation Responses

- Stand one leg-length away, and give personal space.
- Always have an exit available.
- Get assistance (security, panic button).

## TENSION REDUCTION

Once the environment is controlled, reassure individuals that they will receive quality care.

### *FAST FACTS in a NUTSHELL*

De-escalation resources include:
Crisis Prevention Institute: www.crisisprevention.com
Ten Critical De-escalation Skills: www.populararticles.com/article45613.html

PART

II

# Nursing Essentials

# 3

# Vascular Access and Infection Prevention

## Valerie Aarne Grossman

In this chapter, you will discover:

1. Vascular access options
2. Importance of infection prevention
3. Documentation essentials

## VASCULAR ACCESS

Many patients coming to the radiology setting will need vascular access for the completion of their study. Whether an outpatient, inpatient, or emergency department patient, and whether the patient is coming for an imaging study or a procedure, the radiology nurse must have a firm command of the vascular access cannulizations that a patient may have. The nurse must understand how the combination of technology in radiology can help or hurt the patient.

When utilizing a patient's vascular access for a radiologic purpose, it is required for the nurse to be completely familiar with the manufacturer's guidelines for that product (peripheral intravenous [PIV] line, central venous catheter (CVC), intraosseous line, power injection, contrast essentials, and so on), governing entities (organizational policies, State Nurse Practice Act, Food and Drug Administration [FDA] regulations, The Joint Commission), as well as professional organizations (Infusion Nurses Society, Association of periOperative Registered Nurses [AORN], Association for Radiologic & Imaging Nursing [ARIN], American College of Radiology, and so on).

- PIV catheter
  - Recognize the size of the catheter needed to safely perform the study.
  - Verify placement and optimal functioning of the catheter prior to use.
  - Common sizes for use are 18 gauge, 20 gauge, or 22 gauge.
  - Common sites are the distal upper extremity (antecubital fossa is preferred; American College of Radiology, 2013a).
    - When performing a power injection, **avoid** PIVs that are placed in areas of flexion, feet, hands, or external jugular (Infusion Nurses Society, 2011).
- Central venous catheter
  - Must follow manufacturer's recommendations for safe use
  - Must verify patency and follow strict infection prevention steps
  - Understand the interaction of the CVC with the power injector and with the contrast being injected: ultimately, understand how it affects the patient and the imaging (Grossman, 2012)
- Intraosseous vascular access
  - Increasing in popularity among emergency response teams (inside of hospitals as well as in prehospital care)
  - Emerging research regarding safe practice of computed tomography (CT) contrast injection (Aarne Grossman, 2013a)

Regardless of the modality a patient visits within a radiology setting, the patient should be provided with an environment that is, among other essentials, free from infection transmission. This takes the diligence of all who work within that modality to have in place a routine process that guarantees constant cleanliness. Most health care–associated infections occur due to a contaminated surface: a table surface, IV line port surface, procedural table equipment surface, or the surface of a human body. Members of the radiology team, regardless of modality, must use critical observation when ensuring the cleanliness of their work area and patient care area: The responsibility rests upon the shoulders of all team members! Essential steps include:

- Use meticulous hand hygiene
  - At the beginning and end of each work shift
  - Before and after each patient contact
  - Before and after taking breaks
  - Before and after using the restroom
  - After removing gloves (as well as personal protection equipment [PPE])
- Use standard precautions for all patients at all times
  - Follow organizational policies for infection prevention of equipment, tables, IV lines, and for prohibiting the spread of infection in any direction.
- Use additional precautions (PPE) for known higher risk of cross contamination (patients with tuberculosis, *Clostridium difficile* [C-Diff], and so on).
- Adequate equipment cleaning and disinfecting after each patient use, and label as clean
  - Know which cleaning product should be used on which surface without damaging the piece of equipment (Association of periOperative Registered Nurses, 2012).
- Policies should be in place and followed to minimize the risk of contamination, including prohibiting workplace activities such as:
  - Eating
  - Drinking
  - Smoking
  - Applying makeup or lip balm
  - Handling contact lenses

- Procedural rooms should follow current guidelines from all governing agencies, professional organizations, and their own organization's policies.

## FAST FACTS in a NUTSHELL

Refer to the excellent, jointly authored document entitled "Joint Practice Guideline for Sterile Technique during Vascular and Interventional Radiology Procedures" by the Society of Interventional Radiology, AORN, and ARIN, which is also endorsed by the Cardiovascular and Interventional Radiology Society of Europe and the Canadian Interventional Radiology Association (www.sirweb.org/clinical/cpg/QI35.pdf) (Chan, Downing, Keough, Saad, & Annamalai, 2012).

# 4

# ECG Basics

## Andrew Mangiacapre

In this chapter, you will discover:

1. Basic cardiac anatomy and electrophysiology review
2. Fundamental steps in electrocardiogram (ECG) interpretation
3. Importance of comparing a clinical picture to an ECG rhythm strip

## CARDIAC TELEMETRY MONITORING FOR THE RADIOLOGY PATIENT

Electrocardiograph technology is a widely implemented assessment and monitoring tool used in the care of both nonacute and acute care patients, and is quickly becoming an assessment *standard of care*. Nurses working in environments with telemetry monitoring are required to maintain proficiency in understanding and identifying basic cardiac rhythms. The increase in use of monitoring is driven by a commitment to reduce morbidity and mortality associated with arrhythmia. Patients undergoing radiologic procedures commonly receive this monitoring.

The radiology nurse cares for a patient population that spans a spectrum of illnesses and disease pathologies that require ECG monitoring and assessment. In interventional radiology (IR), the practice of a "least-invasive" approach to diagnoses and treatment with the use of wires and catheters possesses increased risk for potentiating and exacerbating underlying arrhythmias. The depth of assessment acumen and skill must parallel our patient population. We owe it to our patients to maintain an ongoing commitment to education and best-practice initiatives. The following is meant as a review of basic knowledge that can be applied in a variety of clinical settings where cardiac monitoring is required.

## FUNDAMENTALS OF CARDIAC MONITORING AND INTRODUCTORY INTERPRETATION

The fundamental principles of the ECG as it is represented on the ECG graph paper include amplitude (voltage), time, foci, and pattern: It traces the low-voltage electrical impulses relative to their energy, timing, location of origin, and regularity. What the ECG *cannot* provide is information as to the heart's ability to pump blood, cardiac remodeling resulting from injury, or cardiac output. This information requires additional diagnostic modalities. It is therefore important to recognize that the ECG has little relevance as a stand-alone diagnostic tool, and priority must be focused upon the patient's clinical presentation.

## *FAST FACTS in a NUTSHELL*

Three strategies to successful ECG interpretation are:

1. Assess, assess, assess (your patient's clinical presentation).
2. Know your Ps and QRSs.
3. "Stripping the patient," which simply translates to putting the patient and strip together for an understanding of the cardiac event or activity taking place.

## CARDIAC ANATOMY AND PHYSIOLOGY

The heart is composed of cardiac-specific:

- **Myocardial muscle cells**
  - These cells contain the contractile filaments actin and myosin, construct the muscle of the atria and ventricles,

and require an organized electrical stimulus to contract effectively.

- **Specialized pacemaker cells**
  - Their primary function is to generate and conduct electrical impulses.
  - They are capable of automatically generating their own electrical impulse (automaticity) absent of any external stimuli.
  - These cells control rate and rhythm and are located in the electrical conduction system of the heart, specifically in the:
    - Sinoatrial (SA) node
    - Atrioventricular junction
    - Bundle of His (BOH)
    - Purkinje network

Other essential intrinsic features of pacer cells are the cell's ability to conduct and transmit electrical impulses (conductivity) and respond to electrical stimuli (irritability). These are important clinical features to understand, particularly when considering the effects of cell hypoxia, electrolyte derangement, and drug toxicity as common causes of dysrhythmias and often encountered comorbidities familiar to the radiology setting. End-stage renal disease, coronary thrombosis, vascular disease, and sedation all carry a component that can alter myocyte cell irritability and action potential threshold propagating dysrhythmia.

## REVIEW OF CONDUCTION PATHWAYS AND COMMON PACERS

The heart is comprised of three essential pacing pathways, allowing for the conduction of stimulus synchronously throughout the heart chambers. These essential pacers include the SA node, AV node, BOH, and Purkinje network. Each pair of chambers has its own pacer rates with characteristic morphology as conduction occurs through each chamber of the heart and is graphed on the ECG rhythm strip. The characteristic "footprint" of each component of the ECG, that is, P, QRS, and T waves, enables rapid interpretation of origin of the stimulus (foci) and/or aberrancy in conduction patterns.

Initial stimulus begins in the SA node, located in the right atrium, that travels down interconnected tracts between nodes called internodal pathways. These pathways are superhighways for transmission of electrical stimulus to each of the chambers, initiating a contraction. A delay of approximately .05 second allows for complete emptying of blood out of the atrium and into the ventricle before tricuspid valve closure. This is known as "atrial kick" and is an important feature of conduction.

## ECG GRAPH PAPER FUNDAMENTALS

The graph paper is arranged with a series of small and large boxes on a horizontal axis relating to time and a vertical axis for measurement of voltage. The horizontal axis will be significant in the interpretation of rate, rhythm, regularity, and time interval between phases of polarization (resting) and depolarization (contraction) of atria and ventricles.

This illustrates a 6-second tracing of a normal-appearing ECG:

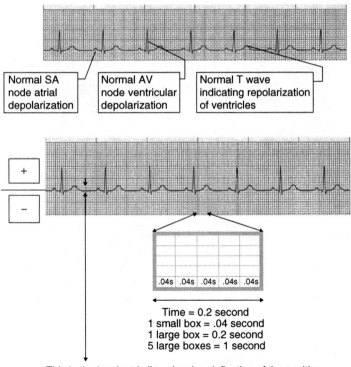

| Normal SA node atrial depolarization | Normal AV node ventricular depolarization | Normal T wave indicating repolarization of ventricles |

.04s .04s .04s .04s .04s

Time = 0.2 second
1 small box = .04 second
1 large box = 0.2 second
5 large boxes = 1 second

This is the isoelectric line showing deflection of the positive and negative energy as it passes through the myocardium.

When interpreting an ECG rhythm strip, remember these important steps:

- **Consider the present state of the patient**
  - STEM = Situation, Treatment, Event, Medications
- **Rhythm**
  - Identify if there are P waves followed by QRS complexes. If yes, then it is normal sinus rhythm [NSR].
  - Do the P $\rightarrow$ P and the R $\rightarrow$ R complexes "march out" regularly? If yes, then is it NSR.
- **Rate** (will identify the node location initiating the impulse)
  - SA node: 60 to 100 beats per minute (bpm)
  - Atrioventricular node: 40 to 60 bpm
  - Ventricular rate: 20 to 40 bpm
- **Direction of the P waves**
  - Upright = sinus rhythm
  - Inverted = junctional escape
- **QRS complex width**
  - Normal: SA ($\leq$ .12 sec)
  - Narrow: Junctional rhythm
  - Wide: Ventricular ($>$ .12 sec)
- **P $\rightarrow$ R interval**
  - Normal interval = .12 sec $\rightarrow$ .20 sec (if lengthened, consider heart blocks)

## *FAST FACTS in a NUTSHELL*

Index cards or the backside of ECG paper flipped up on itself can make for a handy caliper.

# 5

# ECG Rhythm Strips

Andrew Mangiacapre

In this chapter, you will discover:

The different cardiac rhythms
- Sinus rhythms
- Atrial rhythms
- Ventricular rhythms

## SINUS RHYTHMS

### Normal Sinus Rhythm

Appearance: normal; rate: 80; rhythm: regular; P wave: present; QRS: normal < .12; PR interval [PRI]: .20

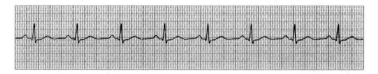

- Impulse conduction:
  - Primary pacemaker sinoatrial [SA] down internodal pathway to atrioventricular [AV] node
  - Normal impulse delay then to ventricles

- Possible causes:
  - Stable patient
  - Unstable, unresponsive, pulseless patient: Consider pulseless electrical activity

## Sinus Bradycardia

Appearance: normal; rate: 40; rhythm: regular; P wave: present; QRS: normal < .12; PRI: 0.20

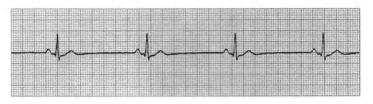

- Impulse conduction:
  - Normal impulse originates from SA node.
  - Conduction is slow across nodal pathway to ventricles, resulting in decreased heart rate of < 60 beats per minute (BPM).
- Possible causes:
  - Increased parasympathetic tone
  - Athletic
  - Drug toxicity (consider digoxin, calcium channel blockers, beta blockers, or narcotics)
  - Vomiting
  - Rest
  - Hypothermia
  - Myocardial infarction
- Significance:
  - No prognostic significance in otherwise healthy subjects
  - May cause dizziness, hypotension, or syncope
- Management:
  - Atropine if symptomatic

## Sinus Tachycardia

Rate: > 100; rhythm: regular; P wave is identical before each QRS; PRI: normal; QRS: normal

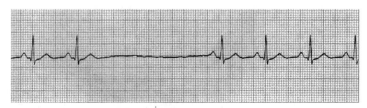

- Impulse conduction:
  - Each beat originates in the sinus node; however, impulse formation in the SA node increases, resulting in a faster heart rate.
  - Each beat is conducted normally through the AV node to the ventricles.
- Possible causes:
  - Exercise
  - Fever
  - Anxiety
  - Pain
  - Caffeine
  - Hypovolemia
  - Hypoxia
  - Ischemia
  - Bronchodilators
  - Congestive heart failure
  - Pulmonary embolus
  - Myocardial infarction
  - Excess stimulants
- Significance:
  - Can affect cardiac output.
  - Ventricular filling time is decreased, resulting in decreased perfusion.
  - Increases cardiac workload.
- Management:
  - Treat underlying cause.
  - Continue to monitor.
  - Consider beta blockers, calcium channel blockers, fluids, or analgesics.

## Sinus Arrest

Appearance: abnormal rate: 60; P wave: present; QRS: normal < .12; PRI: .20

- Impulse conduction:
  - SA node fails to initiate an impulse, causing an absence of one or more PQRST intervals on the rhythm strip, but the rest of the rhythm appears as normal sinus.
- Possible causes:
  - Digoxin
  - Salicylates
  - Hypoxia
  - Ischemia
  - Myocardial infarction
- Significance:
  - May cause dizziness or alterations in consciousness.
- Management:
  - If stable, continue monitoring the patient.
  - If unstable patient, treat the cause.

## ATRIAL DYSRHYTHMIAS

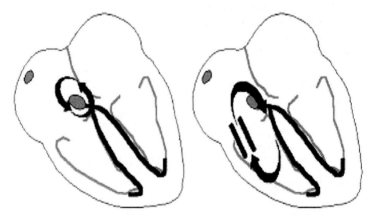

### Origin of Atrial Rhythms

- If SA node fails to initiate an impulse, the surrounding atrial tissue will initiate an impulse from a single ectopic or multiple foci within the atria and internodal pathway.
- Impulses can then be conducted via accessory pathways, which become direct routes from the AV node to the ventricles, skipping the SA node and sinus pathways.

# Atrial Flutter

Rate: atrial 250 to 350, ventricular < 300; rhythm: regular or variable; P wave: saw-toothed flutter waves; QRS: normal

- Impulse conduction:
  - The AV node is the gatekeeper, and based on the number of atrial impulses it gets it will regulate the ventricular response.
  - Atrial flutter with a ventricular rate > 100 BPM is considered an A-flutter with rapid ventricular response.
- Possible causes:
  - Hypoxia
  - Digoxin toxicity
  - Congestive heart failure
  - Myocardial infarction
  - Coronary artery disease
  - Hypertension
  - Chronic obstructive pulmonary disease
  - Status post open heart surgery
  - Pulmonary embolus
  - Cardiac valvular disease
- Significance:
  - May cause palpitations, dyspnea, chest discomfort, syncope.
  - May promote clot formation from slowing the circulating blood.
- Management:
  - Anticoagulant therapy
  - Cardioversion
  - Calcium channel blockers
  - Beta blockers
  - Ablation

## Atrial Fibrillation

Rate: atrial 350 to 700, ventricular slow to rapid rate; rhythm: irregular; P wave: fibrillations; PRI: N/A; QRS: normal but do not march out regularly in rate

- Impulse conduction:
  - The regular cardiac electrical impulses that are normally generated by the sinoatrial node are overwhelmed by disorganized electrical impulses usually originating in the roots of the pulmonary veins. This leads to irregular conduction of impulses to the ventricles, which generate the heartbeat and, thus, result in atrial fibrillation.
- Possible causes:
  - Myocardial infarction
  - Elderly
  - Chronic obstructive pulmonary disease
  - Coronary artery disease
  - Atrial septal defect
  - Mitral valve prolapse
- Significance:
  - Atria quiver and are therefore unable to completely empty, which results in blood stasis, clot formation, and the need for anticoagulation.
  - Decreased cardiac output
  - Loss of atrial kick
  - Leading cause of thrombotic strokes
  - May cause cerebral or pulmonary embolism
- Management:
  - Quinine
  - Digoxin
  - Anticoagulation
  - Synchronized cardioversion, if unstable

## FAST FACTS in a NUTSHELL

Artifact can often be misread as atrial fibrillation (A-Fib). The difference is that artifact typically has QRS R-R regularity and A-Fib has the appearance of "scribble" with an irregular R-R complex.

# Atrial Supraventricular Tachycardia

Rate: 130 to 250; rhythm: regular or slightly irregular; P wave: absent or buried; PRI: N/A; QRS: normal

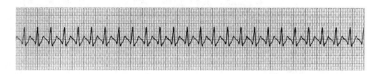

- Impulse conduction:
  - An irritable focus within the atria fires and initiates a rapid re-entrant rhythm within the AV junction, which overrides the sinus node for control of the heart.
- Possible causes:
  - Anxiety
  - Hyperthyroidism
  - Cocaine
  - Caffeine
  - Bronchodilators
  - Alcohol intoxication
  - Energy drinks
  - Anxiety
  - Stimulants
- Significance:
  - May cause palpitations, dyspnea, chest pain, and/or dizziness.
- Management:
  - Vagal maneuvers (bend over, pinch nose, and blow out, and so on)
  - Oxygen
  - Adenosine rapid intravenous (IV) push, in IV closest to the heart (can cause transient asystole)
  - Synchronized cardioversion (refractory supraventricular tachycardia)
    - If cardioverting, make sure to select "synchronization" button and look for R-wave hash marks on screen to prevent deadly "R-on-T."
  - Rate and rhythm can also be paroxysmal.

## Junctional Rhythms

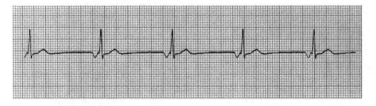

- Impulse conduction:
  - SA node fails and AV node becomes backup pacer.
  - Ventricular conduction is normal.
  - Conduction pathway escapes past junction toward atrium, classic inverted P-wave "junctional escape."
  - Retrograde P wave would appear after QRS.
- Possible causes:
  - Increase vagal tone
  - Myocardial infarction
  - Hypoxia
- Significance:
  - Decreased cardiac output, hypotension, dizziness, and/or syncope
- Management:
  - Atropine
  - Pacing if symptomatic

## VENTRICULAR DYSRHYTHMIAS

### Premature Ventricular Complex (PVC)

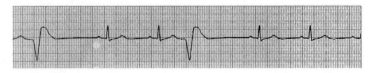

- Impulse conduction:
  - Impulses come from lower ventricular muscle and travel up the ventricles, causing wide QRS pattern ≥ .12 sec (3 or more small boxes).
  - PVCs are complexes, not "contractions," as they do not move blood around.
  - No P waves

- Possible causes:
  - Hypoxia
  - Drug toxicity
  - Hyperkalemia (commonly seen in end-stage renal disease)
  - Irritable foci from the presence of an interventional wire passing through the ventricle
- Significance:
  - No blood is circulated through the heart.
  - Ventricular pacing rate 20 to 40 bpm.
  - > 6 PVC/min produces a danger of converting to lethal dysrhythmias.
  - More volatile dysrhythmias can deteriorate quickly.
  - Hallmark signs of myocardial irritability.
- Management:
  - Eliminate cause (tobacco, caffeine, wire in the ventricle).
  - Beta blockers and/or calcium channel blockers
  - Antiarrhythmic medications

## Display of Multifocal PVCs, Bigeminy

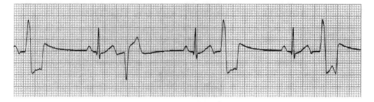

## Display of Multifocal PVCs, Trigeminy

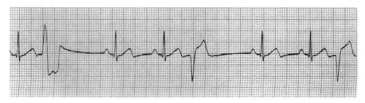

## Monomorphic Ventricular Tachycardia

Ventricular rate: > 150; rhythm: regular; P wave: absent; PRI: N/A; QRS: wide

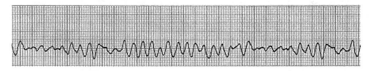

## Ventricular Fibrillation

Rate: N/A; rhythm: chaotic; P wave: absent; PRI: N/A; QRS: indeterminate

# 6

# Sedation and Monitoring

### Lora K. Ott

In this chapter, you will discover:

1. Types of monitoring equipment and purposes
2. Types of procedural sedation and analgesia
3. Recovery process and interventions

## SEDATION AND MONITORING

Intrahospital transport of intensive care unit (ICU) patient guidelines have been established by the Society of Critical Care Medicine and the American College of Critical Care Medicine (Table 6.1). The guidelines require five levels of consideration to be satisfied in order to maintain ICU-level care and monitoring for critically ill patients while in the radiology department.

## TABLE 6.1 Intrahospital Transport of ICU Patient Guidelines

| Patient Needs | Nursing Actions |
| --- | --- |
| Preplanning | Coordination and communication with the ICU staff<br>• Decrease any waiting time in the radiology department<br>• Decrease disruption of the patient's treatments<br>Establish appropriateness of the procedure<br>• Need for contrast<br>• Need for the exam outweighs the risk of transport out of the ICU<br>Scheduling appropriate personnel<br>• Respiratory therapist<br>• ICU-level RN<br>• Critical care medicine physician, if needed<br>Establish procedural risks<br>• MRI screening<br>• Life-supporting intravenous drips<br>• Ability of patient to lie flat, remain still, hold breath<br>Contrast dye allergies<br>• Scheduling contrast premedication<br>• Appropriate IV access |
| Personnel | Minimum of two people trained in intrahospital transport<br>• Minimum of one person certified in resuscitation<br>• ICU-trained RN<br>• Respiratory therapy for all ventilated patients<br>• Physician for all unstable patients |
| Equipment | Equipment to maintain ICU level of care<br>• Transport monitors, including invasive monitoring<br>• Ventilators and airway management<br>• Drug infusions with properly maintained equipment<br>• Identify location crash carts en route to the radiology department |
| Monitoring | Maintain the same level of physiologic monitoring as was being delivered in the ICU<br>• Blood pressure<br>• Pulse oximetry<br>• Cardiac monitoring<br>• Arterial lines |
| Documentation | Maintain a record of patient data<br>• Vital signs<br>• Procedures<br>• Medications<br>• Patient response |

ICU, intensive care unit; IV, intravenous; MRI, magnetic resonance imaging.
Adapted from Warren et al. (2004).

There are no national guidelines established for the transport of non–critically ill acute care patients (non-ICU). However, the ICU guidelines can be applied to the non-ICU patients.

## PROCEDURAL SEDATION AND ANALGESIA

Goals/Purpose—Procedural sedation and analgesia (PSA) allow patients to tolerate painful procedures or procedures that require immobility without undergoing the risks of general anesthesia. Patients undergoing procedural sedation should be able to respond to verbal commands and tactile stimulation. Sedation can be categorized into four levels. The goals for PSA are to provide an altered level of consciousness or anxiety, elevation of pain threshold with possible amnesia of unpleasant events while maintaining a protected airway, stable blood pressure and heart rate, and return the patient to the presedation state prior to discharge. The radiology RN is responsible for administering minimal and moderate sedation to achieve these goals (Table 6.2).

### Preparation for PSA

- Safe administration of PSA requires the proper preparation before any medications are administered (see Table 6.3).

#### Preprocedural Evaluation by the Physician

- A current history and physical, which includes past medical history, review of systems, allergies, and medications, and an airway assessment should be done by a physician.
- The physical examination and vital signs should be updated just prior to the sedation.
- A physician should assign an American Society of Anesthesiologists (ASA) score based on the patient's general health. See Table 6.4 for ASA scores and descriptions.

**TABLE 6.2 Levels of Sedation**

| Level of Sedation | Response to Verbal and Tactile Stimuli | Maintains Airway | Spontaneous Ventilation | Maintains Heart Rate and Blood Pressure |
|---|---|---|---|---|
| Minimal (anxiolysis) | Normal | Yes | Yes | Yes |
| Moderate (conscious) | Purposeful | Yes | Yes | Usually |
| Deep | Repeated verbal and/or painful stimuli required | May require intervention | May be inadequate | Usually |
| General anesthesia | Unresponsive to painful stimuli | Often requires intervention | Often inadequate | May be impaired |

Adapted from Meyers and Chaudhuri (2011).

## TABLE 6.3 Patient Preparation for Procedural Sedation and Analgesia

| Action | Details |
| --- | --- |
| Consent | Informed consent obtained by the physician after being informed of the risks, benefits, limitations, and possible alternatives to procedural sedation. |
| NPO | Fasting guidelines allow for adequate gastric emptying; 2 h for clear liquids, 6 h for a light meal, 8 h for a regular meal. |
| Intravenous access | Intravenous access should be maintained throughout the procedure, until the patient is no longer at risk for cardiovascular or respiratory depression. |
| Supplemental oxygen | Oxygenation via nasal cannula or an alternative appropriate delivery system to decrease the risk of hypoxia during moderate sedation. Recommended by the ASA for all patients receiving moderate sedation. |
| Emergency equipment/ room preparation | Monitoring equipment, suctioning and oxygen delivery equipment are present and in good working order. Resuscitation drugs and fluids, defibrillator, intubation supplies, Ambu bag, and mask are readily available. |
| Personnel | One ACLS-trained person is designated responsible for sedation. |

ACLS, advanced cardiac life support; ASA, American Society of Anesthesiologists; NPO, nothing by mouth.
Adapted from Meyers and Chaudhuri (2011).

## TABLE 6.4 American Society of Anesthesiologists Score

| ASA Level | Description | Risk |
| --- | --- | --- |
| 1 | Healthy patient | Low |
| 2 | Mild systemic disease | Low |
| 3 | Severe systemic disease | High |
| 4 | Severe systemic disease that threatens life | High |
| 5 | Dying patient not expected to survive without procedure | High |
| 6 | Brain-dead patient for organ harvesting for donation | n/a |
| E | Designates the procedure as an emergency | High |

## Monitoring

In addition to respiratory suppression, the medications used for PSA may suppress the autonomic nervous system's ability to adequately respond to hypovolemia; therefore, close monitoring of vital signs is important for the well-being of patients. Refer to Table 6.5 for the recommended monitoring types and intervals, refer to Table 6.6 for the common anxiolytic medications used during procedures, and refer to Table 6.7 for the common analgesic medications used during procedures.

## FAST FACTS in a NUTSHELL

- An informed patient is more cooperative and needs less sedation.
- Sedation cannot make up for poor technique.
- "Less is more": It is easier and safer to add smaller doses than to reverse what has already been given.

PSA medication that may be used in the radiology department by ICU-level staff or with increased training can be found in Table 6.8.

## Postrecovery Care and Discharge

PSA medications promote a rapid recovery stage with minimal postprocedure impairment. The recovery and discharge process will be institution specific. Patients need to be observed until there is no risk of cardiorespiratory depression or compromise; monitoring vital signs, including level of consciousness (LOC), with ability to intervene quickly with resuscitation efforts if needed. An ACLS-trained nurse needs to attend to the recovery process until the patient is stable, meeting the discharge criteria set by the individual institution. Examples of discharge criteria are the Aldrete Scoring System and the Postanesthesia Discharge Scoring System (see Table 6.9).

Prior to discharge the patients should be:

- Alert, oriented, and at baseline
- Discharged with a responsible adult who can be the designated driver, assume care for the patient, and recognize and communicate complications

**TABLE 6.5 Monitoring Types and Intervals**

| Monitored Vital Sign | Method | Frequency | Rationale |
|---|---|---|---|
| Level of consciousness | Provide verbal or tactile stimuli | Prior to administration, repeated doses of medications | Best indicator of sedation effect, best indicator of patient's ability to protect airway |
| Oxygenation | Pulse oximetry | Continuous | Early identification of hypoxia |
| Ventilation | Respiratory rate, capnography for moderate and deep sedation | Every 5 min, continuous with capnography | Direct observation of frequency and quality of respiratory effort |
| Circulation | Heart rate, blood pressure, ECG monitoring | Every 5 min, heart rate and blood pressure; ECG continuous | Early recognition of hypovolemia |
| Temperature | Oral and skin temperature | Once prior to, during, and after procedure | Identification of temperature fluctuations |
| Level of sedation (see Table 6.2) | 0–None<br>1–Minimal<br>2–Moderate<br>3–Deep sedation<br>4–General anesthesia | Every 5 min | To prevent oversedation and early identification of the need for emergency intervention |

ECG, electrocardiogram.

## TABLE 6.6 Most Commonly Used Medications by Radiology Nurses for Sedation

| Generic (Trade) Sedation/Anxiolytics | Dosing | Onset | Duration | Nursing Considerations |
|---|---|---|---|---|
| *Moderate* | | | | |
| midazolam | IV bolus: 1–2.5 mg over 2–5 min. May repeat 25% of initial dose prn, total dose of > 5 mg rarely needed | 1.5–5 min | 2–6 hours | Previously known by the trade name Versed, give slow IV push, rapid infusion may cause hypotension, titrate dose carefully to avoid hypoventilation and hypoxemia, effect perpetuated by the use of opioids |
| *Mild* | | | | |
| diazepam (Valium) | IV: 2–10 mg over 1–5 min, may repeat in 3–4 hours. PO: 2–10 mg 2–4 times/24 hours | IV: 1–5 min. PO: 30–60 min | IV: 15–60 min. PO: up to 24 hours | Anxiolysis effects, decreases muscle spasms and seizure activity, potentiates the effects of opioids, record baseline vital signs prior to administration, known to cause phlebitis and venous thrombosis at IV site, not stable with other drugs |
| lorazepam (Ativan) | IV: 0.044 mg/kg not to exceed 2 mg over 2–5 min. PO: 1–3 mg 2–3 times/24 hours | IV: 15–30 min. PO: 15–60 min | IV: 8–12 hours. PO: 8–12 hours | Anxiolysis effects, IV administration rate not to exceed 2 mg/min or 0.05 mg/kg over 2–5 min, rapid infusion has been known to cause hypotension, apnea, bradycardia, and cardiac arrest, dilute lorazepam 1:1 with normal saline for IV use |
| **Reversal Agent—Benzodiazepine/Antagonist** | | | | |
| flumazenil (Romazicon) | IV: 0.2 mg repeated at 1-min intervals, max. dose = 1 mg. May repeat regime every 20 min, not to exceed 3 mg/hours | 1–2 min | 30–60 min | A competitive antagonist at the receptor site, metabolized by the liver, reliably reverses the amnesia, sedation, and respiratory depression of benzodiazepines associated with nausea and vomiting, seizures when benzodiazepine used for seizure control, and increased sympathetic tone following its administration |

IV, intravenous; PO, by mouth; prn = as needed.
Adapted from Meyers and Chaudhuri (2011); Vallerand and Sanoski (2012).

**TABLE 6.7 Commonly Used Medications by Radiology Nurses for Analgesia**

| Generic (Trade) Analgesia | Dosing | Onset | Duration | Nursing Considerations |
|---|---|---|---|---|
| **Moderate** | | | | |
| fentanyl (Sublimaze) | Bolus: 25–100 mcg over 1–3 min<br>May repeat 25 mcg every 3 min | 1–2 min<br>Peak: 3–5 min | 30–60 min | Rapid onset and shorter duration of action, respiratory depressant effect may last longer than the analgesia, used in combination with midazolam |
| *Pain management* | | | | |
| hydromorphone (Dilaudid) | IV: 1.5 mg every 3–4 hours initially, dose may need to be increased slowly over 2 min | 10–15 min | 2–3 hours | Not commonly used in combination with anxiolytics, do not confuse with morphine, slow IV push, rapid infusion may cause respiratory depression and hypotension, assess respiratory status |
| morphine | IV: 4–10 mg every 3–4 hours, over 5 min | Rapid | 4–5 hours | Not commonly used in combination with anxiolytics, administer 2.5–15 mg over 5 min to avoid respiratory depression and hypotension |
| **Reversal Agent—Opioid/Antagonist** | | | | |
| naloxone | IV: 0.4 mg, may repeat every 2–3 min, max. dose = 2 mg<br>Dilute in 10 cc sterile water or 0.9% NaCl, give over 2 min | 1–2 min | 45 min | Rapid removal from the brain; short duration of action, one dose typically only lasts 30–45 min; repeated doses may be necessary; increased sympathetic tone may occur, manifested as tachycardia, hypertension, pulmonary edema, and cardiac arrhythmias such as ventricular fibrillation |

IV, intravenous; NaCl, sodium chloride.
Adapted from Meyers and Chaudhuri (2011); Vallerand and Sanoski (2012).

## TABLE 6.8 Advanced PSA Medications

| Medication | Description of Action |
|---|---|
| sufentanil (Sufenta) | 5 to 15 times more potent than fentanyl, used as an adjunct for anesthesia or epidural, administered as a bolus dose of 0.1 mcg/kg, side effects of bradycardia and hypotension, not dose dependent, airway management required |
| alfentanil (Alfenta) | One fifth to one tenth as potent as fentanyl, rapid onset 1-4 min, shorter duration than fentanyl, strong respiratory depression |
| propofol (Diprivan) | Short-acting intravenous anesthetic agent with a milky white appearance, used as a hypnotic for sedation purposes, no analgesic effects, potentiates the effects of opioids and benzodiazepines, is not a reversal agent, should only be administered by providers trained in its use and able to manage the potentially life-threatening side effects of hypotension and respiratory depression/apnea, endotracheal intubation equipment readily available |
| methohexital (Brevital) | Onset of action of less than 1 min, with duration of action of less than 10 min; sedative-hypnotic agent with no analgesic effects; produces unconscious state with frequently preserved airway reflexes; side effects of hypotension, hypoventilation, and hypoxemia |
| ketamine | Rapid onset of effect; produces excellent analgesia and amnesia; used as an adjunct to propofol for procedural sedation; minimal respiratory depression; use can be associated with unpleasant psychomimetic effects, such as hallucinations, vivid dreams, out-of-body and distorted visual and auditory sensations; may cause elevation blood pressure, heart rate, and cardiac output, increased oral-pharyngeal secretions |
| etomidate (Amidate) | sedative-hypnotic that lacks analgesic effect, rapid onset of action (less than 1 min), duration of action of 3–5 min, may potentiate seizures |
| dexmedetomidine (Precedex) | Hypnotic and analgesic properties, sedation more closely resembles physiologic sleep, to be used with intubated and mechanically ventilated patients, currently only approved for ICU sedation; however, several studies have demonstrated its utility for sedation outside of the critical care setting |
| nitrous oxide | $N_2O$ is both colorless and odorless and has analgesic and anxiolytic properties, likelihood of moderate to deep sedation increases with the use of other sedating or analgesic medications, causes cardiopulmonary depression in high concentrations, oxygen needs to be administered at all times with the ability to supply 100% oxygen, increased risk of nausea and vomiting |

ICU, intensive care unit.
Adapted from Meyers and Chaudhuri (2011); Vallerand and Sanoski (2012).

## TABLE 6.9 Postprocedure Recovery Score

**Postanesthesia Discharge Scoring System**

Vital signs
Within 20% of preoperative values — 2
20%–40% — 1
40% — 0

Activity/mental status
Oriented and steady gait — 2
Oriented or steady gait — 1
Neither — 0

Pain, nausea, emesis
Minimal — 2
Moderate — 1
Severe — 0

Bleeding
Minimal — 2
Moderate — 1
Severe — 0

Intake and output
PO fluids and voided — 2
PO fluids or voided — 1
Neither — 0

Score ≥ 9 needed for safe discharge to home

**Aldrete Scoring System**

Activity: Able to move, voluntarily or on command
Four extremities — 2
Two extremities — 1
No extremities — 0

Respiration
Able to breathe deeply and cough freely — 2
Dyspnea, swallow or irritated breathing — 1
Apneic — 0

Circulation
BP +/- 20 mmHg of pre-PSA level — 2
BP +/- 20-49 mmHg of pre-PSA level — 1
BP +50 mmHg of preoperative level — 0

Consciousness
Fully awake — 2
Arousable on calling — 1
Unresponsive — 0

Oxygen saturation
Normal, pink — 2
Pale, dusky, blotchy — 1
Cyanotic — 0

Score ≥ 9 points required for recovery confirmed

BP, blood pressure; PO, by mouth; PSA, procedural sedation and analgesia.
Adapted from Meyers and Chaudhuri (2011).

- Provided written discharge instructions, follow-up care and emergency contact numbers
- Provided a signed copy of the discharge instructions for the medical record

## Rapid Response System (RRS)

The RRS provides critical care expertise when ICU-level care is needed for compromised patients outside of the ICU, including radiology. The RRS is the radiology nurse's resource when patients have adverse reactions to sedation, procedures, or diagnostic tests (see Tables 6.10 and 6.11).

| TABLE 6.10 Causes for RRS Deployment in Radiology |
|---|
| • Cardiovascular compromise: hypotension, arrhythmia, chest pain, fluid overload |
| • Respiratory distress: shortness of breath, pulmonary emboli, pulmonary edema |
| • Neurologic events: altered LOC, stroke, seizure |
| • Trauma: falls from scanning table during transfer, dislodged lines, chest tubes |
| • Anaphylaxis: adverse reactions to contrast dye and medications |
| • ICU patients requiring ICU-level intervention while outside ICU environment |

ICU, intensive care unit; LOC, level of consciousness; RRS, rapid response system.
*Source:* Ott et al. (2012).

## TABLE 6.11 Radiology Nurses' Responsibility to the RRS

- Know the institution's RRS call criteria; post and make visible to all staff
- Continual surveillance of sedation patients facilitates rapid RRS deployment
- Nonsedation radiology patients also at risk for requiring the RRS, identify patients at greatest risk for compromise for rapid RRS deployment should call criteria be met
- Participate with the RRS, providing history of care and events prior to the RRS call
- Record and document RRS call, treatments, and outcomes
- Keep the patient and family informed of what is taking place and why

ICU, intensive care unit; RRS, rapid response system.

*FAST FACTS in a NUTSHELL*

Call the RRS when patients meet call criteria—*delay jeopardizes patient safety.*

# 7

# Documentation

## Brooke Grandusky-Green

In this chapter, you will discover:

1. The purpose of electronic medical records
2. Terminology associated with electronic documentation
3. Integration of patient care with electronic documentation

In the nursing profession there is an old saying, "If you didn't document it then it wasn't done." Nurses working in a fast-paced radiology environment must have the skills to document clearly and concisely the timeline of care delivered and the patient's response to the care. The radiology nurse's documentation is essential to capture the "story" of the interventional radiology procedure or assist the provider in what to include in the dictation of the exam report. Furthermore, the radiology nurse needs to document timely assessments and assume the care of the patient while away from the emergency department (ED) or inpatient unit, or while in a procedural/imaging area.

Because of federal legislation, much of the documentation done in patient care settings will now be electronic. Electronic health records (EHRs) are designed so that documentation is easier and more standardized. EHR documentation also provides valuable tools for reporting data and improving care. Clinicians are able to access patient data across a variety of situations, such as in the ED, inpatient, and ambulatory settings. EHR documentation has opened up many opportunities to improve documentation and communication among the radiology department and primary care team. Hand-off reports can be done in person, with a phone call, as well as with a computerized report, and radiology nurses can document on the same medication administration record. The EHR supports both the inpatient and ambulatory care providers in accessing image links as well as the preliminary and final reports. A previous disconnect between imaging records and medical records existed, but with an EHR there can now be "one chart."

## FAST FACTS in a NUTSHELL

The changes that are forthcoming in the health care world further stress the importance of accurate and complete documentation. Payment for expensive diagnostic tests will depend on the documentation supporting the necessity of the exam. While the bedside RN may not see the implications of omitting information or rushing through a health history, patients may feel the impact when they get a bill for services denied. The information that we document not only helps guide the care of the patient, but it also justifies the necessity of the care.

If the picture archiving and communication system (PACS) and radiology information system (RIS) are separate, then it is imperative that there are thoughtful decisions on how to best document care of the patient while in radiology. Departmental workflows and customized documentation tools are very important. Clinical staff should be deeply involved in the building of the EHR as well as making decisions about how the EHR should be used at the bedside. The diverse modalities in radiology may add EHR documentation challenges for the nurse. For example, the nurse in computed tomography (CT) documents differently from the nurse in MRI. The interventional radiology nurse sedates/monitors patients and the nurse in nuclear medicine may need to assist with the injecting of radiopharmaceuticals into a central venous catheter. All actions are different, and the radiology nurse will need an EHR system that will allow proper documentation of the nursing care delivered.

Much of the documentation in a radiology setting may be captured in an electronic format, while some departments may still use paper for some actions. There are many terms associated with the documentation of information that pertain to the EHR and radiology itself.

- RIS
  - Information systems, usually computer-assisted, designed to store, manipulate, and retrieve information for planning, organizing, directing, and controlling administrative activities associated with the provision and utilization of radiology services and facilities (MedConditions, 2013).
- PACS
  - Imaging technology used to store and access images from multiple modalities
  - Replaces film with electronically stored and displayed digital images
- Electronic medical record (EMR)
  - Digital version of a paper chart that contains all of a patient's medical history from one practice
  - Mostly used by providers for diagnosis and treatment (healthit.gov)
- EHR
  - Includes a more comprehensive patient history and is designed to contain and share information from all providers involved in a patient's care
  - Allows patient health to move with them (healthit.gov)
- Meaningful use (MU)
  - Set of standards defined by the Centers for Medicare & Medicaid Services (CMS) Incentive Programs that govern the use of EHRs and allow eligible providers/hospitals to earn incentive payments by meeting specific criteria (healthit.gov)
  - Goal of MU is to promote the use of EHRs and improve health care
- Health Insurance Portability and Accountability Act of 1996 (HIPAA)
  - Protects the privacy of the patient's health information, regulates the security of electronically protected health

information, mandates notification following a breach in the security of protected health information, and ensures the protection of identifiable information, which may be used to analyze patient safety events and improve patient safety
- Best Practice Advisory (BPA)
  - Communicate updates regarding a method or technique that has consistently shown results superior to those achieved with other means
- Health Information Technology for Economic and Clinical Health (HITECH) Act enacted as part of the American Recovery and Reinvestment Act of 2009 and signed into law on February 17, 2009, to promote the adoption and meaningful use of health information technology
  - Subtitle D of the HITECH Act addresses the privacy and security concerns associated with the electronic transmission of health information, in part through several provisions that strengthen the civil and criminal enforcement of the HIPAA rules (www.hhs.gov/ocr/privacy/hipaa/administrative/enforcementrule/hitechenforcementifr.html).
- ARRA: The American Recovery and Reinvestment Act of 2009
- HIMSS: Healthcare Information and Management Systems Society
- ICD-10-CM/PCS: *International Classification of Diseases, 10th Edition,* Clinical Modification/Procedure Coding System. ICD-10 diagnosis codes were created by the World Health Organization and are used to report medical diagnoses and inpatient procedures.
- CMS: Agency within the U.S. Department of Health and Human Services that oversees many key federal health care programs including EHR incentive programs, MU, HIPAA, Medicare, and Medicaid.

Successful documentation in radiology depends on several components, including:
  - Support of senior leadership
  - Attention to detail and impact of documentation upon workflows
  - Adequate resources to document appropriately (time, equipment)
  - Documentation standards in place to guide staff

The EHR is a *tool* utilized to document care delivered. Thus, staff need 24/7 access to technical support and enough computers to document patient care. Although documentation in health care is essential, no tool should ever distract a staff member from the purpose of his or her work. Never lose sight that the patient in front of you is a human being who deserves your utmost compassion and attention.

7. DOCUMENTATION

# Radiologic Imaging Modalities: CT and MRI

# 8

# Computed Axial Tomography Basics

## Valerie Aarne Grossman

In this chapter, you will discover:

1. Basic information regarding the computed tomography (CT) scanner
2. Patient preparation for a CT scan
3. Essential patient education

Computed axial tomography (CAT), or CT, scan is a relatively "young" modality, having first been discussed in the 1970s. The technology uses computer-processed x-rays to create slices (i.e., tomographic images) of a specific body part. The early CT scanners took up to 20 minutes per scan, could only scan the head (which had to be surrounded by a bag of water to reduce the range of dynamic x-rays), and could take hours to process the information for the radiologist to read (Beckmann, 2006). In a mere 40 years of practice, CT scans have progressed to the current 3-dimensional (3D) images, take only minutes to obtain, can scan any body part or organ, and have 64- to 356-slice capability. CT scans are further enhanced with the use of different contrast media that localize to particular image cuts, highlighting images for the interpreting radiologist.

## *FAST FACTS in a NUTSHELL*

The higher the "slice number" of a CT scanner, the thinner is the horizontal picture. For example, a 64-slice CT scanner will take twice the number of pictures as a 32-slice scanner, providing a greater number of images for the radiologist and making it possible to identify even smaller pathology before it grows larger.

CT scans have grown in popularity over the years, with approximately 85 million being done annually in the United States and 63 million in Japan (Brenner, 2012; International Marketing Ventures, 2012; Tsushima, Taketomi-Takahashi, Takei, Otake, & Endo, 2010), although in the United Kingdom the average number of annual CT scans is a mere 3.4 million. The continued growth in use of this technology in the United States is fueled by the ever-present demand to decrease emergency department (ED) overcrowding and the demand for a quick path to diagnosis, faster implementation of treatment, reduced time in radiology and EDs, and facilitation of hospital admission. Virtual colonoscopies and oncology treatment planning also add to the increased use of this technology.

When a patient comes to us for a scan, it is important to remember this event from the patient's perspective. It is always a time of stress for the patient, regardless if he or she is an outpatient (often pending a difficult diagnosis and already worried about the impact such bad news would have on his or her family), an inpatient (scan results could mean complication of a hospital course), or an ED patient (does acute abdominal pain mean the patient will need surgery?). It is rare that a patient comes to the CT scanner without an element of extreme worry about what the scan may reveal and ultimately mean for his or her state of health. The nurse caring for this patient must focus on the "patient behind the image" and guide each patient through the experience. Provide for the patient's privacy, utilize therapeutic touch, make eye contact, and listen to what is being said (or *not* being said). This will ultimately make the experience less stressful for the patient, provide better images for the technologist, and facilitate a more accurate patient assessment for the nurse.

Each CT table has a weight limit and a bore girth limit. To maintain patient dignity, weigh and measure the patient prior to placing patient onto the CT table. When moving large patients, mobilize additional staff to assist and employ professional sensitivity, as large patients often worry about falling from skinny tables or not fitting into small places. Treat the patient with respect and educate the patient regarding your decision-making process.

## SCREENING

An accurate and thorough patient assessment is essential prior to each CT scan. Even if the patient had a recent scan, a thorough patient assessment should take place prior to each and every CT scan. Individual organizational policy will dictate what should be reviewed during the patient history and how the scan procedure may be altered based on information obtained during the patient prescan assessment. Conditions that may be considered follow.

### Allergies

- A history of prior anaphylactic reaction to an allergen may place the patient at a higher risk of reacting to CT contrast media.
- Shellfish/seafood allergy does NOT predispose a patient to a contrast media allergy.
- A prior allergic reaction to contrast media is a serious finding and needs careful attention before the patient receives contrast in the future (see the Premedication section in Chapter 10).

### Anxiety

- Provide a calm environment for all patients and educate them about each step of the scan process, as it is imperative for patients to be motionless during the CT scan.
- Caregivers must be professional and convey competence to their patients.

# Asthma

- Consider listening to breath sounds and identifying when the patient last used a rescue inhaler.
- There may be an increased risk of intravenous (IV) contrast reaction in patients with asthma.

# Breastfeeding

- It is considered safe for breastfeeding mothers to receive contrast, as less than 1% of iodinated contrast media that is administered to a mother is excreted through her breast milk, and less than 1% of the contrast media in breast milk is absorbed into the infant's gastrointestinal tract (American College of Radiology, 2013a).
- Mothers who would like more information can contact the Poison Control Center at (800) 222-1222 for the latest information on contrast media and breastfeeding.

# Cardiac Status

- Care should be taken when administering contrast media to patients with a cardiac history, including angina, hypertension (treated with medication), congestive heart failure, severe aortic stenosis, primary pulmonary hypertension, or cardiomyopathy.
- Decreasing the volume or osmolality of contrast may increase patient safety.
- Refer to "physiological effects of contrast" for more information.

# Devices

- Identify and, if possible, remove metal from the body, as it will create "scatter" on the image: It will distort the images being interpreted by the radiologist.
- Any types of metal in the area of the body to be scanned should be removed (i.e., body piercings, jewelry, hearing aids, and so on).

## Dehydration

- Scans may increase the risk of nephrotoxicity in patients with impaired renal function, multiple myeloma, sickle cell disease, gout, homocystinuria, and so on.
- Blood urea nitrogen (BUN) > 20 mg/dL may indicate the need for hydration before/after receiving IV iodinated contrast medium.

## Hypertension

- Patients who receive medication to treat hypertension are at increased risk of contrast-induced nephrotoxicity.

## Hyperthyroidism

- Graves' disease, Plummer's disease, and toxic adenoma may predispose a patient to thyrotoxicosis 4 to 6 weeks after receiving IV iodinated contrast.

## Metformin

- Metformin is excreted unchanged from the kidneys and causes increased lactic acid production from the intestines. As IV contrast is also excreted through the kidneys, together there is too much workload placed on the kidneys.
- Liver dysfunction, alcohol abuse, cardiac failure, infection, sepsis, or any muscle ischemia increases the risk of lactic acidosis occurring in these patients.
- Patients should be advised to omit metformin from their regime for 48 hours post-IV contrast administration.

## Multiple Myeloma

- May develop irreversible renal failure following administration of high-osmolality contrast media, especially if the patient is dehydrated.

# Pheochromocytoma

- High-osmolality contrast media may increase the serum catecholamine levels and result in hypertensive crisis, while nonionic contrast media may have no influence on serum catecholamine levels (Bessell-Browne & O'Malley, 2007).

# Pregnancy

- Iodinated contrast media crosses the placenta and enters the fetus.
- The physician should thoroughly explain the risk of IV contrast and exposure to CT radiation to the pregnant mother, and informed consent should be signed prior to the procedure.

# Renal Insufficiency

- An increased serum creatinine level (> 1.3 mg/dL) or decreased glomerular filtration rate (< 59 mL/min) may indicate risk for contrast-induced nephrotoxicity (CIN).
- Lab work should be within 24 hours for the typical inpatient or ED patient, while some organizations use the 4- to 6-week time period for lab values with outpatients. This practice varies among organizations.
- Emergent situations (stroke, trauma, and so on) may necessitate obtaining a CT scan without waiting for lab results, per your organization's policy.
- Predisposing factors for CIN could include:
  - Age > 60 years old
  - History of renal disease
    - Dialysis (should occur within 24 hours of CT contrast)
    - Kidney transplant
    - Single kidney
    - Renal cancer
    - Renal surgery
    - Proteinuria
  - Diabetes mellitus
  - Taking a medication containing metformin (used to treat diabetes; may also be used by some physicians in the treatment of polycystic ovarian disease)

- Dehydration (BUN > 20 mg/dL)
- Hypertension (receiving medication for treatment)
- Multiple contrast studies in less than a 24- to 48-hour period

## Sickle Cell Disease

- There is some belief that IV contrast can promote sickle cell crisis.

## PATIENT EDUCATION

Educating the patient who is having a CT scan should begin the moment you introduce yourself to the patient and explain your role in his or her care. For some, this may be their first experience having a CT scan, or perhaps their first experience with a particular type of contrast. Help them to feel welcome and safe in your department. Explain what you are going to do BEFORE you do it. Take the time to answer their questions, and involve patients in their care as much as possible.

- It is important to teach your patients about:
  - Scan table and scanner
    - Movement of the table and scanner
    - Breath-holding instructions
    - The proper position to be in during the scan
    - That staff can see them, even though he or she is alone in the room
  - Injection
    - Purpose of IV contrast
    - Position of extremity (with peripheral IV placed)
    - Possible sensation that occurs during injection
  - Post-scan
    - Seek advice from the ordering physician regarding avoidance of metformin-containing medications for 48 hours post-contrast injection
    - Importance of hydration post-contrast (if received IV contrast)
    - Possibility of mild gastrointestinal symptoms (if received oral contrast)
    - Call 911 for respiratory distress or a medical emergency

    – Contact the ordering physician for mild allergic-type reactions up to 7 days post-IV contrast
    – Explain when results will be interpreted by the radiologist

## SPECIAL CONSIDERATIONS

CT technology is also useful in other areas of health care, such as dentistry, virtual colonography, radiation therapy, positron emission tomography (PET) scans, and areas outside of health care where industrial CT scanning may assist in fields such as museum artifact conservation, engineering applications, and metrology.

- Dental CT scans provide 3D images that are used in special situations such as diagnosing pathology, tumors, or surgical planning.
- Virtual CT colonoscopy has less risk, less cost, and is less invasive than a conventional colonoscopy, although it does expose the patient to radiation. If pathology is identified the patient will need to undergo a conventional colonoscopy for treatment.
- PET scans are nuclear medicine scans and CT scans that are superimposed on each other. They provide the radiologist with images that identify molecular activity within the body as well as interpretable images.

# 9

# Iodinated Contrast (CT) Media Basics

## Valerie Aarne Grossman

In this chapter, you will discover:

1. Screening of a patient prior to receiving contrast
2. Different types of contrast media
3. Physiologic effects of intravenous (IV) iodinated contrast

## CONTRAST

The use of contrast media enhances the images being read by the radiologist and leads to a more accurate identification of internal structures and pathology. Contrast can be used in a variety of different ways and is available in many different types. Each modality within the radiology setting has contrast types that are used for specific studies. Common types of contrast for computed tomography (CT) scans are:

- Oral
  - Barium sulfate
    - Micro pulverized white powder that comes in various forms.
    - Concentration mixture varies with the exam being done.
    - Volume of contrast used depends on the procedure, anatomy, and transit time.
    - 1,000 to 2,000 mL is needed for the average colon study.
  - Iodinated water-soluble contrast
    - High-osmolar contrast media (HOCM) are water soluble and hypertonic.
    - Diluted with water for CT scans.
  - Water
    - Plain water may be used as an oral contrast for certain exams.
- Rectal
  - Iodinated water-soluble contrast mixed with water, given via enema just prior to scanning.
- IV iodinated contrast media
  - Injected through a patent IV line, it opacifies the vessels in its flow path, allowing the visualization of internal structures until significant hemodilution occurs. The contrast media subsequently flows toward the extravascular compartments, where it is absorbed by normal and abnormal tissues in the body and the brain. Finally, it is excreted unchanged through the kidney by glomerular filtration. The degree of density enhancement is directly related to the content of iodine, the dose used, and the rate of injection.
  - Three primary forms of contrast exist:
    - HOCM, the oldest agents, have limited use.
    - Low-osmolar contrast media (LOCM) is water soluble and most commonly used.
    - Nonionic or iso-osmolar contrast media (IOCM) is not water soluble.
  - IV CT contrast should be warmed to body temperature prior to administration, as it will then decrease the viscosity and promote a safer injection.
  - Verify patency of IV lines (peripheral or central) by following manufacturer and organization policy (venous backflow, easily flushes, painless insertion site, visual image of central venous catheter tip, and so on)

To prevent an air embolism, perform a double safety check when connecting the tubing from the power injector to the patient's IV: Survey the entire length of the tubing with your eyes, observing for air just prior to connecting the injector tubing to the patient's IV line, and look for a drop of contrast protruding from the tip of the tubing.

## PHYSIOLOGIC EFFECTS OF IODINATED CONTRAST INJECTION

- **Cardiac effects following IV CT contrast injection**
  - "Hot flash" sensation is common from vasodilation
  - Depression of the sinoatrial automaticity, causing bradycardia or even sinus arrest
  - Transient heart block due to depression of the atrioventricular node
  - Hypotension due to decreased contractility of the heart muscle
  - Disturbances in electrical conduction (with ionic contrasts)
  - Cardiac output may increase due to systemic vasodilation and increased intravascular volume
- **Cerebral effects following IV contrast injection**
  - Bradycardia due to carotid stimulation
  - Systemic hypotension post injection of carotid or vertebral arteries from stimulating the pressure sensors on the vessels and the vasomotor activation in the brain
  - "Warmth" or pain in the face due to dilation of the external carotid artery
  - Nausea and vomiting may occur when contrast crosses the blood–brain barrier
- **Gastrointestinal tract effects following IV contrast injection**
  - Nausea, vomiting, diarrhea, or cramping
  - Some patients may "taste" a metallic flavor
  - Pancreatic swelling leading to pancreatitis
  - Swelling of the salivary glands leading to parotitis
- **Peripheral vascular effects following IV contrast injection**
  - Vasodilation and "warmth" at site
  - Local vascular spasm can occur, which can initially be painful for the patient
  - Pain can occur due to red blood cell (RBC) crenation

- **Pheochromocytoma effects following IV contrast injection**
  - This is a rare neoplasm of adrenal gland tissue that results in the release of too much epinephrine and norepinephrine.
  - HOCM can induce a hypertensive crisis as well as hyperadrenergic symptoms (anxiety, tremors, agitation, nausea).
  - LOCM has not been shown to have this same effect.
- **Pulmonary effects following IV contrast injection**
  - von Bezold-Jarisch reflex can occur, resulting in bradycardia, hypotension, hypopnea, and peripheral vasodilation.
  - Bronchoconstriction may occur due to histamine release, as contrast is seen as a foreign body in the bloodstream.
- **Renal effects following IV contrast injection**
  - Patients with diabetes and preexisting renal insufficiency are at greatest risk of nephrotoxicity.
  - Increased risk of contrast-induced nephrotoxicity (CIN) in patients who have received contrast within the previous 24 to 48 hours.
  - Healthy kidneys will excrete contrast in 2 to 4 hours; impaired kidneys (reduced glomerular filtration rate [eGFR], elevated creatinine, elevated blood urea nitrogen [BUN]) may take several days to excrete contrast.
  - It can take up to a week for serum creatinine to return to normal after a patient receives IV contrast.

$\Rightarrow$ Protect your patient's kidneys by carefully reviewing his or her eGFR (should be $> 59$ mL/min/1.73 m$^2$) and BUN (normal is 6 to 20 mg/dL).

## FAST FACTS in a NUTSHELL

Anuric end-stage chronic kidney disease patients can receive IV iodinated contrast, as their kidneys are no longer functioning and it will be cleared with dialysis. Emergent dialysis is not necessary, though some recommend dialysis within 24 hours of contrast injection. Care should be taken with oliguric patients, as there is a belief they may be converted to anuric patients after receiving IV iodinated contrast media.

- **Thyroid effects following IV contrast injection**
  - Iodine in contrast agents can stimulate an acute overproduction of thyroid hormone in patients with an occult or

overt hyperthyroid condition, such as Graves' disease, hyperactive nodule, thyroid adenoma, toxic multinodular goiter (Plummer's disease).

- Administer CT contrast with care in these patients; recommend follow-up with their endocrinologist after receiving IV contrast.
- Jod-Basedow syndrome is a delayed thyroid storm that occurs after the administration of iodinated CT contrast (Carroll & Matfin, 2010).

- **Vascular effects following IV contrast injection**
  - Fluid shifts from the tissues to the veins because contrast has higher osmolality than blood (contrast is heavier than blood, so fluid from cells goes back into the veins to thin out the blood).
  - Peripheral vasodilation, especially at the injection site (patient may initially feel a "burn" when injection begins, which calms down after a few seconds).
  - Transient blood pressure drop occurs (approximately 30 to 45 seconds) because of the fluid shift.
  - Reflex tachycardia occurs because of vasodilation (vessel membranes open up to promote movement of fluids).
  - Vasodilation may make the patient feel "warmth" or a "hot flash" with the injection.
  - Care should be taken with compromised patients, including those with aortic stenosis and severe coronary artery disease, among others.
  - RBCs shrink because the water is removed from the cell to help balance blood plasma-contrast solution.
    - This crenation (dehydration) of RBCs causes their shape to change, creating an inability to float through the capillary with ease, and ultimately decreases oxygenation to the tissues. This can be harmful to patients with sickle cell anemia.
    - Thrombosis or ischemia may occur, especially in the brain or myocardium.
  - Vascular endothelial damage could occur, as the contrast can be toxic to the tissue.
    - When damage occurs to the inside lumen of the blood vessel, the risk of a blood clot occurs due to the activation of the clotting cascade (Robbins & Pozniak, 2010).

Power injectors force contrast through the body at precision speed to be expertly timed with the radiation scanning of the CT. It is important for the nurse performing the injection to remember the equivalent injection rates of the power injector:

(Power injector rate)  1 mL/sec is equivalent to 3,600 mL/hr    (IV pump rate)
2 mL/sec is equivalent to 7,200 mL/hr
3 mL/sec is equivalent to 10,800 mL/hr
4 mL/sec is equivalent to 14,400 mL/hr
5 mL/sec is equivalent to 18,000 mL/hr

## PREINJECTION VERIFICATION ("TIME OUT")

Prior to each injection of contrast, the organization must have a policy to STOP and double check all vital indicators for the patient about to be scanned. Included in this "time out" verification at minimum should be:

- Two patient identifiers
- Review of the provider's order for scan
- Proper scan on the correct body region and laterality
- Need for scout films
- Allergies and other risks reconciled
- Correct contrast, dose, concentration, and rate of injection
- How much of a delay between injection and start of scan? Can the nurse stay with the patient for the entire injection?

It is essential for the nurse or the technologist who performs the injection to STOP and double check that all steps have been safely completed before approving the start of the contrast injection.

## PATIENT EDUCATION

As detailed also in Chapter 8, educating the patient who is having a CT scan should begin the moment you introduce yourself to the patient and explain your role in his or her care. For some patients, this may be their first experience having a CT scan, or perhaps their first experience with a particular type of contrast. Help them to feel welcome and safe in your department. Explain what you are going to do BEFORE you do it. Take the time to answer their questions, and involve patients in their care as much as possible.

- It is important to teach your patients about:
  - Scan table and scanner
    - Movement of the table and scanner
    - Breath-holding instructions
    - The proper position to be in during the scan
    - That staff can see them, even though he or she is alone in the room
  - Injection
    - Purpose of IV contrast
    - Position of extremity (with peripheral IV placed)
    - Possible sensation that occurs during injection
      - "Hot flash" anywhere from their throat, stomach, genital region
      - May feel as though they are urinating on themselves
  - Post-scan
    - Seek advice from the ordering physician regarding avoidance of metformin-containing medications for 48 hours post-contrast injection.
    - Importance of hydration post-contrast (if received IV contrast).
    - Possibility of mild gastrointestinal (GI) symptoms (if received oral contrast) or headache following IV contrast.
    - Call 911 for respiratory distress or a medical emergency.
    - Contact primary care provider or ordering physician for mild allergic-type reactions up to 7 days post-IV contrast.
    - Explain when results will be interpreted by the radiologist.

# 10

# Iodinated Contrast (CT) Adverse Events

## Valerie Aarne Grossman

In this chapter, you will discover:

1. Emergency treatment of reaction
2. Treatment of extravasation
3. Pretreatment for prior contrast reactions

## IODINATED CONTRAST ADVERSE EVENTS

The risks associated with CT contrast have diminished over the years as the contents have changed and the understanding of their use has improved. Patients have become informed consumers and often protect themselves from unnecessary exposure to the risks of contrast studies. From intravenous (IV) extravasation to allergic reactions, there are steps that are vital to follow for safe patient care in the computed axial tomography (CAT) scan setting.

Allergic IV CT contrast reactions may occur immediately or be delayed by up to 7 days. Typically, the more severe the reaction, the quicker the symptoms will begin. If your patient begins to exhibit symptoms before the scan is complete, the nurse in attendance should mobilize a response team immediately, as the patient is likely to progress to anaphylaxis quickly!

Patients may experience a wide variety of contrast events that may require observation, treatment, and education.

## Mild Reactions

- Signs and symptoms appear self-limited without evidence of progression
- Allergic signs or symptoms include:
  - Urticaria/pruritis
  - Cutaneous edema
  - Itchy or scratchy throat
  - Nasal congestion
  - Sneezing, conjunctivitis, rhinorrhea
- Physiologic signs or symptoms include:
  - Nausea or vomiting
  - Transient flushing, warmth, chills
  - Headache, dizziness, anxiety, altered taste
  - Mild hypertension
  - Vasovagal reaction, which resolves without treatment

## Moderate Reactions

- Signs and symptoms are more pronounced and require medical management.
- May progress to a more severe reaction if treatment is delayed.
- Allergic signs or symptoms include:
  - Diffuse urticaria or pruritis
  - Diffuse erythema with stable vital signs
  - Facial edema without dyspnea
  - Throat tightness or hoarseness without dyspnea
  - Wheezing or bronchospasm with mild or no hypoxia
- Physiologic reactions:
  - Protracted nausea or vomiting
  - Hypertensive urgency
  - Isolated chest pain
  - Vasovagal reaction that responds to required treatment

## Severe Reactions

- Signs and symptoms are often life-threatening and may result in permanent injury or death if not managed immediately and appropriately.
- Patient condition may quickly progress to cardiopulmonary arrest.

- Pulmonary edema, although rare, can occur in patients with impaired cardiac function.
- Allergic life-threatening reactions:
  - Diffuse edema with or without facial edema causing dyspnea
  - Diffuse erythema with hypotension
  - Laryngeal edema with stridor and/or hypoxia
  - Wheezing or bronchospasm with significant hypoxia
  - Anaphylactic shock with hypotension and tachycardia
- Physiologic life-threatening reactions:
  - Vasovagal reaction resistant to treatment
  - Arrhythmia
  - Seizure
  - Hypertensive crisis

## Reaction Management

- If you suspect a patient is having a reaction, do NOT remove the IV (you may need it later!).
- Call for additional personnel to assist, and perform a rapid patient assessment with vital signs.
- Interventions will depend upon your patient's signs and symptoms, but could include the following:
  - Monitor vital signs (heart rate, respiratory rate, blood pressure, oximetry, capnography, electrocardiogram, and so on).
  - Access patient medical history, medication list, allergies, weight.
  - IV fluids (hypotension, anaphylaxis, hypoglycemia).
  - Administer oxygen (bronchospasm, laryngeal edema, hypotension/hypertension, pulmonary edema, seizures).
- Position for rescue
  - Elevate the head of the bed (dyspnea, pulmonary edema)
  - Trendelenburg (hypotension)
  - Position patient on his or her side (seizures)
- Medications for treatment may include:
  - Diphenhydramine (hives)
  - Epinephrine (progressive hives, diffuse erythema, bronchospasm, laryngeal edema)
  - Beta agonist inhaler (bronchospasm)
  - Atropine (hypotension, bradycardia)
  - Labetalol (hypertension)
  - Nitroglycerin (hypertension)
  - Furosemide (hypertension, pulmonary edema)

- Morphine (pulmonary edema)
- Lorazepam (seizures)
- Dextrose 50% (hypoglycemia)
- Glucagon (hypoglycemia)

Refer to current advanced cardiac life support (ACLS) guidelines, rescue protocols, and your organization's policies.

## Allergy Premedication (Iodinated Contrast Media)

For patients who have experienced past adverse reactions with IV iodinated contrast, their physicians will order premedication prior to their receiving iodinated CT contrast. While there are different prescriber preferences regarding the premedication regime, it is important to realize the importance of antihistamines and that the maximum prophylactic benefit of corticosteroids occurs at a minimum of 6 to 13 hours after the first dose is administered. After identifying an "at-risk" patient from a history of prior contrast reaction, the current recommendation from the 2013 American College of Radiology (ACR) Contrast Manual (ACR, 2013b) for premedication regimen is as follows.

### Elective Studies

#### Option #1

1. Prednisone: 50 mg by mouth at 13 hours, 7 hours, and 1 hour before contrast injection
2. Diphenhydramine: 50 mg IV or by mouth 1 hour prior to contrast injection

#### Option #2

1. Methylprednisolone: 32 mg by mouth at 12 hours and 2 hours prior to contrast injection

## FAST FACTS in a NUTSHELL

- IV corticosteroids are not effective when administered less than 4 hours prior to contrast injection.
- Careful blood glucose monitoring should occur in diabetic patients who receive corticosteroids.

### Option #1

1. Methylprednisolone sodium succinate: 40 mg every 4 hours until contrast injection is administered
   - Hydrocortisone sodium succinate 200 mg IV every 4 hours until contrast injection can be substituted for the methylprednisolone
2. Diphenhydramine: 50 mg IV 1 hour prior to contrast injection

### Option #2

(for patients with known allergy to aspirin, nonsteroidal anti-inflammatory drugs, or methylprednisolone)

1. Dexamethasone sodium sulfate 7.5 mg or betamethasone 6 mg IV every 4 hours until contrast injection administered
2. Diphenhydramine: 50 mg IV 1 hour prior to contrast injection

### Option #3

1. Omit steroids
2. Diphenhydramine: 50 mg IV 1 hour prior to contrast injection

## Pediatric Patients

1. Prednisone: 0.5 to 0.7 mg/kg by mouth (up to 50 mg) given 13 hours, 7 hours, and 1 hour prior to contrast injection
2. Diphenhydramine: 1.25 mg/kg by mouth (up to 50 mg) 1 hour prior to contrast injection

# EXTRAVASATION OF IODINATED CONTRAST MEDIA (CT)

Every patient who receives IV contrast is at risk of extravasation; therefore, it is imperative to work diligently to prevent this.

## Prevention of Extravasation

- Optimal IV placement for patient condition (most appropriate gauge, site, and injection rate for the study to be conducted).

- Verify IV patency prior to injection (follow manufacturer and organizational guidelines, which normally include venous back flow, forceful saline flush, central venous catheter visual image of the tip, and so on).
- Patient education of process (keep arm straight and motionless, "hot flash" feeling, and so on).
- Maintain hyper-focus on the patient during actual injection.
  - If you are able to remain in the scan room with the patient, maintain manual contact at the IV insertion site, monitor the thrill, and be prepared to immediately stop the injection if extravasation begins.

## *FAST FACTS in a NUTSHELL*

If you must monitor an IV power injection from the CT control room, keep your eyes on the patient at all times until the injection is complete. In most cases, when an extravasation begins the patient will flinch and curl the fingers or toes in pain before you will hear him or her scream in pain. This gives you advance notice and allows you to stop the injection and minimize the severity of the extravasation.

## Patients Who Are at Increased Risk for Extravasation

- Cannot communicate adequately
  - Elderly
  - Infants or children
  - Patients with altered consciousness
- Are severely ill, injured, debilitated, or uncooperative for any reason
- Have abnormal circulation to the extremity, including:
  - Atherosclerotic peripheral vascular disease
  - Stroke
  - Raynaud's disease
  - Venous thrombosis or insufficiency
  - Arterial insufficiency
  - Compromised venous/lymphatic drainage in the extremity used for IV injection
  - Diabetic vascular disease
  - Radiation therapy

- Extensive surgery in the limb in which the injection will be done (lymph node dissection, vein graft harvesting, and so on)
- Have IV sites in the:
  - Hand
  - Wrist
  - Foot
  - Ankle
- Have IV sites that were:
  - Placed longer than 24 hours ago
  - Difficult to cannulate
  - Placed by an ambulance crew or during a code situation
  - Already used for multiple power injections
  - Placed in the upper arm with ample loose tissue

## Treatment of Extravasation

- There are a variety of methods, with no clear best practice.
- Immediately stop the infusion of the contrast media at the first sign of extravasation.
- Notify the physician/radiologist.
- May attempt to aspirate contrast through IV needle.
- Elevate the affected extremity above the level of the heart to decrease capillary hydrostatic pressure.
- Gently massage the area to distribute the agent and apply **dry**, cold or warm compresses to relieve the pain.
  - Dry, warm compresses may promote vasodilation and improve absorption and blood flow.
  - Dry, cold compresses may relieve pain at the injection site.
- May attempt injection of corticosteroids or hyaluronidase.
- Document in the patient's medical record the following information related to the infiltration:
  - Location (if possible, measure the size and extent and/or girth of the area affected)
  - Type and amount of contrast medium
  - Treatment that was rendered
- Assess the extremity involved for any of the following:
  - Redness
  - Blisters
  - Ulceration
  - Firmness
  - Changes in temperature, movement, or sensation (ACR, 2013b)

- Patients must be given clear instructions for follow-up, which include seeking medical help for the development of ulcers, worsening pain or swelling, change in sensation or circulation.
  - Nurse-to-nurse report (hand-off) should occur for inpatients and emergency department patients after they receive IV contrast for a CT scan and are documented in the patient's medical record.
  - Good nursing practice includes a follow-up call 24 hours post-extravasation to assess the patient's condition and document in the patient's record.

# 11

# MRI Basics and Magnet Safety

## Valerie Aarne Grossman

In this chapter, you will discover:

1. Screening for magnet safety
2. Use of MRI scan technology
3. Essential patient education

## MRI

In 1974, the first patent was obtained for an MRI scanner, and it wasn't until 1977 that the first patient was scanned, although it took nearly 5 hours to produce just one image. (That first MRI scanner is now housed in the Smithsonian Institution.) Fast forward to 2011, where there are 102.7 MRI scans per 1,000 people in the United States, and 97.4 scans per 1,000 people in Turkey every year (Organisation for Economic Co-operation and Development, 2012).

MRI provides an unparalleled view inside the human body by using strong magnetic fields and radio waves that work together to produce cross-sectional images of organs and internal structures of the body. The MRI detects the signal, which varies depending on the water content and local magnetic properties of the particular body part being imaged, and, thus, different tissues or substances can be distinguished from one another in the resulting scan. An electrical current is passed through wires in a coil, which creates a temporary magnetic field around the patient's body. The radio waves are sent and received from within the machine, and these signals are used to produce digital images of the body part being scanned.

## FAST FACTS in a NUTSHELL

Common units of measure for magnets are tesla and gauss (1 tesla = 10,000 gauss). Most MRI magnets used today are 0.5 to 2 tesla (5,000–20,000 gauss). Compare that to the Earth's natural magnetic pull, which is measured at a mere 0.5 gauss!

MRI is valuable for imaging and diagnosing:

- Multiple sclerosis
- Tumors of the pituitary gland, brain, and bone
- Infections of the brain, spine, and joints
- Ligament injuries
- Joint injuries (shoulder, knee, back)
- Tendonitis
- Early stages of strokes
- Cysts

## MAGNET SAFETY AND SCREENING

With the magnetic pull of the MRI being so intense, the MRI personnel must be diligent to protect the safety of those who may come near it. Both paid personnel and visitors must be screened for magnet safety questioning and metal inside or outside the body. The list is extensive and cannot be fully covered in this text; however, a brief overview will be discussed. A person's simple attestation that *he or she is safe to go near the magnet* is not sufficient: Each person must be fully screened for magnet safety prior to admittance to the magnetic resonance (MR) environment (American College of Radiology [ACR], 2013a).

## FAST FACTS in a NUTSHELL

For the latest information on MRI safety and practice guidance, visit: www.mrisafety.com

## Personnel Responsible for Magnet Safety and Screening

- Each organization must have an MR medical director as well as an MR safety director who maintains an updated safety structure for the department. Initial orientation as well as annual competency for those directly involved with MR patient care must include appropriate documentation of education and attendance at a 1-hour live lecture or recorded presentation (ACR, 2013a).
- Staff who provide care for patients near the magnet must be screened for magnet safety and documentation must be maintained. They should be screened for the same safety risks as the patients, and such documentation should be kept on file.
- Prior to entering the MR scanner, staff must remove all metal from their body including:
  - Wallets (containing bank/identification cards with metallic strips)
  - Pagers, cell phones, watches, pens, keys, nail clippers, jewelry, hair decorations
  - Pocket knife, law enforcement weapons, tools
  - Any metal object will become a dangerous item near the magnet!

## Patient Magnet Safety and Screening

- Patients should be screened for magnet safety by two qualified MR personnel prior to routine scans, and by one qualified MR personnel prior to an emergency scan.
- Unconscious patients who have no history available should minimally have orbital x-rays obtained to screen for metal fragments prior to MRI.
- Ask patients the same question in different ways to account for terminology differences, which could uncover a safety hazard for the patient (i.e., pacemaker vs. implanted device).
- Identify if patients have any of the following:
  - Metal objects in the eye (shavings, slivers, and so on)
  - Any type of electronic, mechanical, or magnetic implant
  - Aneurysm clips
  - Cardiac pacemaker or defibrillator
  - Stimulator (bio-stimulator, neuro-stimulator, spinal cord, bone growth, and so on)

- Internal wires or electrodes
- Cochlear or other otologic implant
- Drug-infusion pump (insulin, chemo, pain medicine, and so on)
- Any prosthesis of any kind
- Implanted valves, joints, rods, pins, devices, coils, filters, stents, clips, staples, shunts, springs, wires, mesh, seeds, plates, dental work, and so on
- Metal object (BB, shrapnel, bullet, and so on)
- Vascular access (port, peripherally inserted central catheter, and so on)
- Tissue expander (i.e., breast)
- Removable or permanent dental piece, denture or partial plate
- Electronic monitoring device
- Body piercings or implants
- Wig or hair implants
- Tattoos or permanent makeup (newly placed)
- Intrauterine device, diaphragm, or vaginal pessary
- Hearing aid
- Any piece of anything that the patient was not born with!
- Additionally, the MR staff will need to carefully assess patients who have:
  - Endotracheal or tracheotomy tubes
  - Central lines, Swan-Ganz catheters, arterial line transducers, and so on
  - Foley catheters with a temperature sensor and/or a metal clamp
  - Esophageal or rectal probes
  - Guidewires
- Prior to entering the MR scanner, patients will be asked to:
  - Use the restroom, if necessary
  - Wear earplugs or headphones
  - Remove jewelry, hair decorations, removable denture plates, hearing aids, eyeglasses, watches, pagers, wallets, purses, cell phones, some body piercings, and clothing with metal

## PATIENT HISTORY AND SCREENING

In addition to screening patients for magnet safety, staff must screen patients for medical history, renal issues, and their ability to comply with the MRI procedure. Prior to positioning the patient on the MRI scan table, determine the following:

- Previous MRI scan or other imaging performed
- Concern for claustrophobia (sedation, someone to drive patient home, and so on)
- History of eye injury (when, type, treatment, and so on)
- Current medication list
- Medication allergies (source, reaction, treatment, premedication, and so on)
- Contrast allergies (type of contrast, reaction, and so on)
- History of asthma, respiratory disease, hypertension, cancer, seizures, diabetes, liver disease, renal disease of any type, anemia, sickle cell anemia, among others (determine specifics of each illness)
- Pregnancy screening (last normal menstrual period, pregnancy test results, fertility treatments, and so on)
- Breastfeeding

## PATIENT EDUCATION

Educating the patient who is having an MRI scan should begin the moment you introduce yourself to the patient and explain your role in his or her care. For some, this visit may be their first experience having a MRI scan, or perhaps their first experience with a particular type of contrast.

═══════════════════════════════════════*FAST FACTS in a NUTSHELL*

Help your patients feel welcome and safe in your department. Explain what you are going to do BEFORE you do it. Take the time to answer their questions, and involve patients in their care as much as possible. The more relaxed patients are, the more cooperative they can be, and the better your scan imaging will be!

- It is essential to teach your patients about:
  - Scan table and scanner
    - Importance of earplugs or headphones to protect their hearing from the sound of the MRI scanner in motion
    - Movement of the table and scanner

- Breath-holding instructions
- The proper position to be in during the scan
- That staff can see them, even though he or she is alone in the room
- The importance of the patient role in image acquisition (holding still, following instructions, and so on)
- Injection
  - Purpose of IV contrast
  - Possible sensation that occurs during injection
- Post-scan
  - Explain when results will be interpreted by the radiologist

# 12

# MRI Contrast Media

## Valerie Aarne Grossman

In this chapter, you will discover:

1. Screening of the patient prior to receiving contrast
2. Different types of contrast media
3. Emergency treatment of reaction

## PATIENT HISTORY AND SCREENING

In addition to screening patients for magnet safety, staff must screen patients for medical history, renal issues, and ability to comply with the MRI procedure. Determine:

- Previous MRI scans or other imaging
- Concern for claustrophobia (sedation, someone to drive the patient home, and so on)
- History of eye injury (when, type, treatment, and so on)
- Current medication list
- Medication allergies (source, reaction, treatment, premedication, and so on)
- Contrast allergies (type of contrast, reaction, and so on)
- History of asthma, respiratory disease, hypertension, cancer, seizures, diabetes, liver disease, renal disease of any type,

anemia, sickle cell anemia, among others (determine specifics of each illness)
- Pregnancy screening (last normal menstrual period, pregnancy test results, fertility treatments, and so on)
- Breastfeeding

## CONTRAST

MRI contrast agents work by altering the local magnetic field of the tissue being imaged. Contrast can be used in a body cavity or injected IV. The different types may include:

- Oral
  - Ultra-low dose/dilute barium sulfate (i.e., Volumen)
  - Fruit juice (pineapple, blueberry)
  - Water
  - Methylcellulose
  - Polyethylene glycol (American College of Radiology [ACR], 2013a)
- Endorectal
  - Sonography transmission gel (Kim et al., 2008)
- Vaginal
  - Aqueous gel (Brown, Mattrey, Stamato, & Sirlin, 2005)
- Intravenous (IV)
  - Gadolinium is a paramagnetic metal ion that moves differently within a magnetic field.
  - Gadolinium-based contrast media are administered at room temperature (15–30°C) per manufacturer guidelines and, therefore, should NOT be warmed prior to IV injection.
  - When injecting gadolinium for IV contrast, the same safety steps must be observed as with computed tomography (CT) IV contrast injections (see Chapter 9).
  - Screen the patient for IV gadolinium safety by assessing for:
    - Metabolic acidosis
    - Immunosuppression
    - Liver disease
    - Age > 60 years old
    - Renal disease (acute or chronic)
      - Dialysis
      - Renal surgery (transplant, tumor removal, and so on)
      - One kidney
      - Cancer

- Multiple myeloma
- Systemic lupus erythematosus
- Glomerular filtration rate < 60 mL/min
  - Lab work should be within 48 hours to 6 weeks depending on comorbidities (ACR, 2013a)

## PREINJECTION VERIFICATION ("TIME OUT")

Prior to each injection of contrast, the organization must have a policy to STOP and double check all vital indicators for the patient about to be scanned. This "time out" verification should minimally include:

- Two patient identifiers
- Review of the provider's order for the scan
- Proper scan on the correct body region and laterality
- Allergies and other risks reconciled
- Correct contrast, dose, concentration, and rate of injection

It is essential for the nurse or technologist who performs the injection to STOP and double check that all safety steps have been completed before approving the start of the contrast injection.

## VERIFY IV PATENCY

Verify patency of the IV lines (peripheral or central IV lines) by following the manufacturer's and organization's policies (venous backflow, easily flushes, painless insertion site, visual image of central venous catheter tip, and so on)

═══════════════════════════*FAST FACTS in a NUTSHELL*

To prevent an air embolism, perform a double safety check when connecting the tubing from the power injector to the patient's IV: Survey the entire length of the tubing with your eyes, observing for air just prior to connecting the injector tubing to the patient's IV line, and look for a drop of contrast protruding from the tip of the tubing.

# EXTRAVASATION

Many MRI scans utilize hand-injected IV gadolinium and therefore the risk of extravasation is small, as close monitoring of the injection should prevent most tissue damage from an infiltrate of gadolinium. Even with power injection of gadolinium, the amount of contrast is typically quite small, and the risk of compartment syndrome from an extravasation is low.

## ADVERSE EVENTS DUE TO CONTRAST

- Mild reactions may include:
  - Nausea/vomiting
  - Headache
  - Dizziness
  - Coldness, warmth, or pain at the injection site plus paresthesias
  - Itching
- Allergy
  - Rash
  - Hives
  - Urticaria
  - Bronchospasm
  - Anaphylactoid
    - Treatment is similar to that of CT IV contrast reactions.
    - Be sure to remove the patient from the MRI scanner prior to providing emergency care.
- Nephrogenic systemic fibrosis
  - Poorly functioning kidneys are not able to excrete gadolinium from the body.
  - Patients receiving dialysis appear to have a slightly higher risk.
  - As a result, excessive fibrous tissue begins to grow on the eyes, skin, joints, and internal organs.
  - For more information: www.fda.gov/drugs/drugsafety/ucm223966.htm

## EMERGENCY RESPONSE

If a patient decompensates while in the MRI scanner, magnetic resonance (MR) personnel should immediately **begin emergent medical interventions while the patient is actively being moved** out of the magnet area. A preestablished, magnetically safe, resuscitative area must be designated within the radiology department.

## Reaction Management

- If you suspect a patient is having a reaction, do NOT remove the IV (you may need it later!).
- Call for additional personnel to assist, and perform a rapid patient assessment with vital signs.
- Interventions will depend upon your patient's signs and symptoms, but could include the following:
  - Monitor vital signs (heart rate, respiratory rate, blood pressure, oximetry, capnography, electrocardiogram, and so on)
  - Access patient medical history, medication list, allergies, weight
  - IV fluids (hypotension, anaphylaxis, hypoglycemia)
  - Administer oxygen (bronchospasm, laryngeal edema, hypotension/hypertension, pulmonary edema, seizures)
  - Position for rescue
    - Elevate the head of the bed (dyspnea, pulmonary edema)
    - Trendelenburg (hypotension)
    - Position patient on his or her side (seizures)
- Medications for treatment may include:
  - Diphenhydramine (hives)
  - Epinephrine (progressive hives, diffuse erythema, bronchospasm, laryngeal edema)
  - Beta agonist inhaler (bronchospasm)
  - Atropine (hypotension, bradycardia)
  - Labetalol (hypertension)
  - Nitroglycerin (hypertension)
  - Furosemide (hypertension, pulmonary edema)
  - Morphine (pulmonary edema)
  - Lorazepam (seizures)
  - Dextrose 50% (hypoglycemia)
  - Glucagon (hypoglycemia)

Refer to current advanced cardiac life support (ACLS) guidelines, rescue protocols, and your organizational policies.

# Allergy Premedication

For patients who have experienced past adverse reactions with IV gadolinium, determine which brand and type caused their prior reactions. Their physicians will order premedication prior to their receiving IV gadolinium contrast in the future. While there are different prescriber preferences with the premedication regime, the important detail to remember is that the maximum prophylactic benefit of corticosteroids occurs a minimum of 6 to 13 hours after the first dose is administered. After identifying an "at-risk" patient from a history of prior contrast reaction, the current recommendation from the 2013 ACR Contrast Manual (ACR, 2013b) for premedication regimen is as follows.

## Elective Studies

### Option #1

1. Prednisone: 50 mg by mouth at 13 hours, 7 hours, and 1 hour before contrast injection
2. Diphenhydramine: 50 mg IV or by mouth, 1 hour prior to contrast injection

### Option #2

1. Methylprednisolone: 32 mg by mouth at 12 hours and 2 hours prior to contrast injection
2. Diphenhydramine: 50 mg IV or by mouth 1 hour prior to contrast injection

## FAST FACTS in a NUTSHELL

- IV corticosteroids are not effective when administered less than 4 hours prior to contrast injection.
- Careful blood glucose monitoring should occur in diabetic patients who receive corticosteroids.

## Emergent Studies

### Option #1

1. Methylprednisolone sodium succinate: 40 mg every 4 hours until contrast injection occurs

- Hydrocortisone sodium succinate 200 mg IV every 4 hours until contrast injection can be substituted for the methylprednisolone
2. Diphenhydramine: 50 mg IV 1 hour prior to contrast injection

## Option #2

(for patients with known allergy to aspirin, nonsteroidal anti-inflammatory drugs, or methylprednisolone)

1. Dexamethasone sodium sulfate 7.5 mg or betamethasone 6 mg IV every 4 hours until contrast injection is administered
2. Diphenhydramine: 50 mg IV 1 hour prior to contrast injection

## Option #3

1. Omit steroids
2. Diphenhydramine: 50 mg IV 1 hour prior to contrast injection

### Pediatric Patients

1. Prednisone: 0.5 to 0.7 mg/kg by mouth (up to 50 mg) given 13 hours, 7 hours, and 1 hour prior to contrast injection
2. Diphenhydramine: 1.25 mg/kg by mouth (up to 50 mg) 1 hour prior to contrast injection

## PATIENT EDUCATION

Educating the patient who is having an MRI scan with contrast should begin the moment you introduce yourself to the patient and explain your role in his or her care. For some patients, this may be their first experience having an MRI scan, or perhaps their first experience with a particular type of contrast. Help them to feel welcome and safe in your department. Explain what you are going to do BEFORE you do it. Take the time to answer their questions, and involve patients in their care as much as possible.

- It is important to teach your patients about:
  - Scan table and scanner
    - Importance of earplugs/headphones to protect their hearing from the sound of the MRI scanner in motion

– Movement of the table and scanner
– Breath-holding instructions
– The proper position to be in during the scan
– That staff can see them, even though he or she is alone in the room
– The importance of the patient role in image acquisition (holding still, following instructions, and so on)
- Injection
  – Purpose of IV contrast
  – Possible sensation that occurs during injection
- Post-scan
  – Explain when results will be interpreted by the radiologist

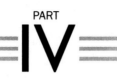

PART

# IV

# Interventional Radiology

# 13

# Neuro-Interventional Radiology Overview

## Susan Deveikis and John P. Deveikis

In this chapter, you will discover:

1. The importance of good communication among all team members
2. The importance of anticipating patient needs before, during, and after procedure
3. The importance of infection control during invasive procedures

## COMMUNICATION

Communication is the key to providing high-quality and safe patient care. Every team member should be aware of the anticipated procedure and his or her role in that procedure. Every team member should feel free to speak up if he or she sees something amiss. The operator (attending physician) should be the most informed person in the room—not the least informed person. The operator is directing all the other team members. For example, anesthesiologists should be aware of their role during intracranial embolization. The anesthetized patient should be made immobile through the use of paralytics and deep sedation, and the anesthesia team should be prepared to do that and to test the anesthetized patient periodically with a nerve stimulator to ensure he or she is adequately paralyzed.

Prior to the procedure, a plan should be in place as to the anticipated disposition of the patient. For example, is the patient going to be an outpatient and has a designated driver? If the patient is to be admitted, will the patient need an intensive care unit (ICU) bed, monitored bed, or just floor status? This information allows the patient to have optimal nursing care postprocedure. Not knowing can lead to lapses in the level of patient care while the location and personnel are being sorted out.

## INFECTION CONTROL

For the best practice, the procedural suites and the neuroangiography suite should base their policy and procedure guidelines for infection control on the recommendations of the Association of periOperative Registered Nurses.

## FAST FACTS in a NUTSHELL

Quality infection control behavior protects both patients and health care workers by preventing personnel from transmitting microorganisms.

All personnel who enter the semirestricted and restricted areas of the angiography suite should wear surgical attire intended for use within the angiography suite. This means the procedural attire should be laundered within the institution.

## FAST FACTS in a NUTSHELL

REMEMBER: *It's all about the patient!*
Be successful in your practice by making your actions better than they have to be:

- Use evidence-based medicine.
- Pay attention to every detail.
- Recognize that "minimally invasive" procedures are still *invasive*.
- Run your angio suite like an operating room.

Hair can collect bacteria when left uncovered and potentially contribute to a wound infection; therefore, it is necessary for hair (head and facial) to be covered at all times. Patients should also wear a surgical cap. All personnel entering restricted areas of the angiography suite should wear a mask when sterile items and equipment are exposed. Masks are intended to contain and filter droplets containing microorganisms that are expelled from the mouth and nasopharynx during talking, sneezing, and coughing. Gloves should be selected and worn, depending on the task to be performed:

- Sterile gloves must be worn for sterile procedures.
- Unsterile gloves may be worn for other tasks, including any encounter with body fluids or potentially infective material.
- Change gloves after each task and between patients to reduce the risk of spread of infection.

## FAST FACTS in a NUTSHELL

University of Michigan study:

- Health care workers with artificial nails are more likely to carry pathogens than those with native nails.
- Artificial nails harbor more bacteria than natural nails, even with scrubbing (www.cdc.gov/ncidod/hip/hand/hhfedreg.htm).
- Avoidance of artificial fingernails or extenders when providing patient care is a Category 1A recommendation.
- Category 1A recommendations are supported by well-designed experimental, clinical, or epidemiologic studies and are strongly recommended.

Hand hygiene and proper use of appropriate barriers such as gowns, gloves, and masks help prevent avoidable infections by potentially drug-resistant pathogens. A surgical scrub should be done prior to setting up the sterile tray. A surgical scrub should be done and a sterile gown and gloves should be worn by the operator and scrub assist. Do not have food in the procedure area; it might attract flies that can spread infection to the procedure room. (It is also torture for a patient who may be fasting to smell food.) All these simple tasks protect the patient from infection. Infection control is important because:

- Infections can adversely affect patient outcome.
- It maintains compliance with organizational infection control policies.

- Infection control is required by The Joint Commission guidelines.
- Hospital-based infections are increasing.
- Hospital-based infections trigger penalties for insurance payments to hospitals.
- Implantation of devices can potentially increase the risk of infection.
- Increased use of closure devices
- Bacteremia can occur in 32% of angiography cases over 2 hours.
- Drug-resistant "super bugs" are now everywhere.

Infection control protects patients and health care workers. Personal protective equipment (hats, masks, gloves, gowns, and face shields) will prevent infective material from patients contaminating the health care worker. Routine hospital laundering of surgical scrubs and *never* wearing hospital scrubs anywhere outside the hospital will help prevent spreading of infective material that may splash or spray during these procedures.

These are the hallmarks of universal precautions:

- Take precautions always, even if you do not suspect dangerous infectious disease.
- Use hats, masks, gloves, gowns, and face shields when performing an invasive procedure.
- Use gloves when handling bodily fluids.

## FAST FACTS in a NUTSHELL

In 1999, New York State signed a law stating that professionals who do not adhere to scientific infection control policies are guilty of unprofessional conduct.

## PATIENT SAFETY

The patient is someone we have been given the privilege and responsibility to treat and protect. His or her life is in our hands. Working as part of a team allows one to ensure high-quality and safe care for patients. Essential to patient safety are:

A. **Patient identification.** This is crucial prior to the start of any procedure. The "time out" procedure should include:
   1. Two patient identifiers (name, date of birth, or medical record number)

2. What procedure is to be done (verify procedural orders, specimen orders, and so on)
3. Consents (procedural, sedation, blood, do not resuscitate [DNR] orders, and so on)
4. Dry-erase board mounted on the wall for key information about the patient and the procedure to provide a quick visual for all members of the team
5. The procedure nurse is responsible for:
   a. Reviewing the patient's neurological status
   b. Baseline vital signs, current lab work, medications, allergies, weight, and medical history
   c. Ensuring documents are in order (consents, electronic documents, and so on)

B. **Hemodynamic monitoring**. This should be conducted on all patients upon admission to the angiography suite and throughout the procedure.
   1. Notify attending physician of any abnormalities.

## FAST FACTS in a NUTSHELL

- All invasive transducers should be attached to the angiography table and zeroed, as the table may be raised and lowered multiple times throughout the procedure.
  - This prevents over/under draining of cerebral spinal fluid from the intracranial pressure (and prevents intracranial crisis).
  - This maintains accurate measurements from arterial lines or central lines.

C. **Medication safety**. This is an area in which the nurse plays an important role.
   1. Drug allergies should be known prior to the procedure and listed on the dry-erase board in the procedure room.
   2. Patient weight in kilograms should be known and also written on the board.
   3. Follow organizational policy to ensure proper medication dosage.
      a. Read labels carefully.
      b. Always double-check doses, and utilize a second nurse to confirm doses for critical medications, like heparin.
   4. Refer to Chapter 6 for more information on procedural sedation and monitoring.

D. **Documentation safety**
1. Routine documentation of vital signs, medications, and patient assessment should be precise throughout the procedure.
2. Documentation of implanted devices (coils, stents, closure devices, and so on) should include the lot number and expiration date.
   a. This could have important implications for the patient's future (MRI compatibility, recall of implanted device, and so on).
3. Refer to Chapter 7 for more information on documentation in the radiology setting.

E. **General safety tips**
1. Smaller is better (very important in babies).
   a. Good rule-of-thumb is to use the smallest groin access possible.
2. Heparin is your friend.
   a. Prevents thrombus on catheter.
3. Label all containers on tray and all syringes (a requirement of The Joint Commission).
4. Empty syringes placed on the sterile procedural table should *never* be full of air.
   a. Either fill the syringes with heparinized saline or contrast.
5. Air bubbles are *not* your friends during neuroangiography.
6. Repetition is your friend.
7. Items can only be either sterile or contaminated: There is no in-between!
8. Eye shields should be worn by all personnel and by the patient during glue embolization due to n-butyl cyanoacrylate (n-BCA).
9. Angiographic (body, cardiac, neurologic) procedures are truly team efforts.
   a. Every team member is essential and everyone has his or her area of expertise.
   b. Everyone must perform at the top of his or her game.
   c. Only when the whole team is patient focused can the institution rise above the ordinary.

Patients should be educated prior to the procedure regarding risks, benefits, and treatment options. Key topics to be thoroughly explained:

A. Preprocedure: Medication information, lab work, appointments, and so forth
   1. The patient should be allowed time to ask any and all questions he or she may have.
B. Intraprocedural:
   1. The patient must be made a team member who is actively involved with getting the procedure accomplished safely and effectively.
   2. Coax the patient to cooperate during key portions of the procedure.
   3. Patients need to be warned in advance that they might feel anything uncomfortable or unexpected.
C. Postprocedural:
   1. Discuss admission expectations or home care.
   2. Advise the patient of what he or she should or shouldn't do, and what symptoms to expect, such as:
      a. It is generally recommended that patients drink plenty of fluids after angiographic procedures.
      b. Patients that have had a closure device placed should not sit in a tub or go swimming for 5 days after procedure.
      c. Most patients may experience some groin tenderness after the local anesthetic wears off, but severe or persistent pain could be a sign of problems like hematoma or infection.
   3. Discuss follow-up appointments.
   4. Provide written instructions prior to discharge.
   5. Be prepared to answer follow-up phone calls if the patient has any question or problems.

*FAST FACTS in a NUTSHELL*

Unanticipated movement during aneurysm coil placement or during n-BCA embolization can be very serious for the patient. Movement may cause the catheter or coil to perforate the aneurysm and may degrade the image during the deposit of n-BCA. Either of these occurrences may lead to a life-threatening scenario.

# PATIENT COMFORT

A professional and clean environment must be maintained at all times. The temperature in the room should be adjusted for patient comfort. A blanket warmer/cooler may be used for optimal temperature regulation for longer cases. Angiography rooms are frequently cold for the comfort of operating personnel wearing hats, masks, gowns, gloves, and lead protection aprons. However, always remember that the patient may be much too cold, which can affect his or her comfort and ability to remain motionless without shivering. It can even have hemodynamic effects on the patient. Other comfort tips:

- The patient's modesty and privacy should be maintained at all times.
- Support and reassurance should be provided to all patients.
- Excess noise, stimulation, and conversation should be kept to a minimum, especially during induction of anesthesia.
- Avoid distracting conversation: The patient should always be the central focus.
  - Laughing and joking heard in the room may make the patient feel uncomfortable and believe that *he or she* is the subject of ridicule, even though it may be an unrelated conversation.
- Do not have food in the procedure area:
  - It is torture for a patient who may be fasting to smell food.
  - Risk of attracting insects.
- Arm and heel supports and padding should be used throughout the procedure to prevent possible ulna nerve and heel damage.
  - The patient's fingers should fit inside the arm supports at all times.
- Foley catheters should be placed with the patient asleep whenever possible.
  - Tape the tubing to the patient's leg with a little slack in the tubing to prevent inadvertent pulling on the catheter. Hang the bag on the side of the angiography table to decrease risk of infection from reflux into the bladder and to accurately measure output.

- Treat each patient as an individual.
- Understand how his or her disease process and the procedure can impact him or her.
- Pay close attention to every detail.
- Only when the whole team is patient focused can the institution rise above the ordinary.

## CRISIS MANAGEMENT

The team should be prepared for a worst-case scenario with each procedure performed. An emergency crash cart and medications must be readily available. Oxygen, suction (make sure suction can reach the length of the angiography table), and appropriately sized Ambu bags, masks, and equipment for intubation must be in the room at all times. The nurse should be familiar with the equipment and know where important items are stored. Point-of-care glucose testing capability should be readily available, especially in diabetic patients that have a sudden change in neurological status. Advanced cardiac life support (ACLS) certification is very important for nurses involved with angiographic procedures and is mandatory for many departments. Be sure that every patient has **two** *functioning* **intravenous lines** (IVs; preferably 18G or larger) and they should be checked for patency prior to groin access. It can be difficult and time-consuming to place the second IV while the patient is crashing. All IV poles and anesthesia equipment should be out of the way of the x-ray equipment. Always have an extra bag of saline available in case you need to give volume in a hurry.

### Emergencies

#### Contrast Reaction

Be sure to check for history of allergies and premedicate patients with a history of contrast allergy. Be suspicious after contrast has been given when the patient shows restlessness, itchiness, or an increased respiratory rate. This could be the first sign of an ana-phylactic reaction. Be prepared to rapidly give oxygen or IV fluids, and have rescue medications available. Refer to Chapter 10 for additional information on iodinated contrast reactions and treatment.

## Aneurysm Rupture

Anticipate a decline in the patient's neurological status. If the patient is not intubated, this may need to be done emergently. If the patient becomes hemodynamically unstable, he or she may need to be supported with volume and blood pressure support. The affected vessel may need to be temporarily shut down with either a balloon or coils emergently. If the patient has a ventriculostomy catheter in place, a rapid change in intracranial pressure may indicate aneurysm rupture and it may be necessary to open the catheter to drain.

## Carotid Angioplasty or Carotid Stenting Crisis

Especially if working with a *de novo* carotid (never had surgery), the patient may develop severe bradycardia and hypotension. Have atropine available. Always have a pacer available and place pacer pads prior to the start of the procedure. Know how to operate the pacer.

## Groin Site Complications

Hematoma can be life-threatening and can threaten the circulation in the affected limb, resulting in amputation. Hematomas can occur even when closure devices are used. Monitoring of the puncture site should be strictly adhered to. Sandbags are not recommended for hematoma because they give a false sense of security. The hematoma goes unrecognized until it expands past the circumference of the bag, allowing greater expansion of the hematoma. Apply a pressure dressing in cases where you might expect hematoma formation, such as elderly patients with friable vessels, patients on anticoagulation, or very obese patients. Excessive groin or back pain should be investigated, since pain can be the first sign of a retroperitoneal bleed or expanding hematoma in the leg. Always check the color, temperature, and distal pulses of the accessed limb to rule out an ischemic problem as well.

# 14

# Neuro-Interventional Procedures

## John P. Deveikis and Susan Deveikis

In this chapter, you will discover:

1. The importance of preparing for complications
2. The importance of rapid stroke care by all team members for improved outcomes
3. The nurse's role in neuro-interventional procedures

The nervous system is vitally important for the normal function of the individual, yet the brain is very sensitive to ischemia. Disorders of vascular supply to the nervous system can have devastating effects on patients and can be fatal. Neuro-interventional procedures are minimally invasive treatments for neurovascular conditions. These procedures can complement or sometimes replace more traditional medical and surgical treatments for these conditions.

# PROCEDURES

A. **Endovascular Ischemic Stroke Treatment**
1. *Description*
   a. Resolution of acute arterial or venous thrombus within a cerebral vessel via catheterization and local infusion of a thrombolytic agent and/or extraction of thrombus.
2. *Indications*
   a. New-onset neurological deficit caused by an acute cerebral thrombus.
3. *Preprocedural workup*
   a. Refer to Table 14.1 for neuro-interventional preprocedural care.
   b. Anticipate intensive care unit (ICU) level of care postprocedure.
   c. Emergency preprocedural evaluation upon arrival to the angiography suite.
   d. Have protamine, heparin, tissue plasminogen activator, nicardipine, and abciximab available at all times.
   e. Anesthesia rarely used.

---

### TABLE 14.1 Neuro-Interventional Preprocedural Care

1. Elective patients will be seen in the preoperative clinic prior to the procedure. Emergency patients' evaluations will be done in the hospital.
2. Nothing by mouth after midnight; consent signed.
3. Identification/consideration of pregnant/nonpregnant state.
4. Obtain assessment, including allergies, neurological status, medical history, current reviewed labs, National Institute of Health (NIH) Stroke Scale (when indicated), recent imaging.
5. Provide patient education/reassurance throughout interactions with patient and family.
6. For outpatients, confirm a designated driver is present before start of procedure.
7. Have patient void (if no Foley catheter).
8. Remove all jewelry and secure per organizational policy.
9. Baseline vital signs and pedal pulses prior to groin puncture.
10. Patent IV(s) (at least 18G or 16G), 0.9% normal saline.
11. Antibiotics may be given.
12. Have suction, Ambu bag, and emergency drugs readily available prior to the patient's arrival.
13. Anticipate postprocedure bed status (when indicated).

---

4. *Intraprocedural care*
   a. Refer to Table 14.2 for neuro-interventional and intra-procedural care.
   b. Conduct frequent neurological assessment and communicate any changes to the attending physician immediately.
   c. Anticipate worst-case scenario, such as cerebral edema or hemorrhage.
   d. Ensure point-of-care coagulation test (activated clotting time) capability.
   e. Prior to recanalization, blood pressure may need to be supported to maximize perfusion. After recanalization, blood pressure may need to be decreased to prevent reperfusion injury and hemorrhage.
   f. Emergent intubation may be necessary depending on the patient's ability to protect his or her airway. Assist anesthesia during emergent intubation or line placement if necessary.
   g. If Foley catheter required, it should be placed using a sterile technique, but *do not delay procedure to place a Foley catheter.*

---

### TABLE 14.2 Neuro-Interventional Intraprocedural Care

1. Verify patient identification upon arrival to angiography suite.
2. Obtain baseline neurological status, monitor for any subtle change in neurological assessment.
3. Never leave patient unattended. Provide emotional support to patient.
4. Place patient on hemodynamic monitors and obtain baseline vital signs. Monitor and record throughout procedure unless performed by anesthesia team.
5. Pad patient's elbows and heels (to prevent skin or nerve damage) and place patient's head in head sponge in a neutral position.
6. Place sequential compression device on bilateral lower extremities.
7. "Time out" prior to groin puncture or per institution policy.
8. If Foley catheter required: Place using sterile technique (after general anesthesia induction) and prior to groin prep and drape.
9. Clip groin according to department infection control policy.
10. Prep and drape in a sterile manner (follow manufacturer's recommendations for drying time of skin prep prior to draping patient).

- Acute stroke **MUST** be treated rapidly.
- Neurons are dying every minute, so any delay can worsen outcome.
- Do not waste time with tasks that can be done later; for example, Foley catheter placement, talking about the next case, and so on.
- This is an *emergency* and the entire team needs to focus on caring for the patient quickly.

    5. *Postprocedural care*
        a. Refer to Table 14.3 for neuro-interventional postprocedural care.
        b. Anticipate ICU postprocedure.
    6. *Follow-up*
        a. May do immediate postprocedure computed tomography (CT) scan if concerned for acute hemorrhage or otherwise routinely done within 24 hours.
        b. Workup for cause of stroke and prevent possible recurrence.
  B. Carotid Stenting
    1. *Description*
        a. Dilation of narrowed segment by inflating a balloon (angioplasty) followed by placement of cylinder mesh to maintain normal vessel caliber and increase blood flow to the brain.

---

### TABLE 14.3 Neuro-Interventional Postprocedural Care

1. Obtain postprocedure pedal pulses. Check groin puncture site upon completion of procedure and then every 15 minutes × 3, every 30 minutes × 2, every 1 hour × 1.
2. Strict bed rest with accessed leg extended for 1 to 2 hours if closure device placed (or 6 hours if no closure device used).
3. Neurological exam upon completion of procedure and then per protocol.
4. Call report to receiving nurse.
5. Accompany patient to receiving department.
6. Unless nothing by mouth (NPO), encourage oral fluids postprocedure, 100 mL over next 4 hours.
7. Resume preprocedure diet and medications as indicated.

2. **Indication**
   a. Symptomatic in spite of maximal medical therapy and not a good candidate for open surgical endarterectomy.
3. **Preprocedural workup**
   a. Refer to Table 14.1 for neuro-interventional preprocedural care.
   b. Anticipate ICU postprocedure.
   c. Antibiotics may be given prior to implantation of stent.
   d. Antiplatelet agents may be loaded immediately prior to procedure or may have been started several days before.
   e. Have heparin, protamine, atropine, and abciximab available at all times.
   f. Usually done without anesthesia.

## FAST FACTS in a NUTSHELL

- Inflation of a balloon at the carotid bifurcation can stimulate the pressure receptors in the vessel wall and result in sudden, often severe, bradycardia and hypotension.
- Worst-case scenario: Patient may become asystolic.
- Mild cases may resolve as soon as balloon is deflated.
- IV atropine may help with persistent bradycardia.
- Be prepared to administer external pacing for severe bradycardia with hypotension.

4. **Intraprocedural care**
   a. Refer to Table 14.2 for neuro-interventional intraprocedural care.
   b. Place temporary pacer pads on patient prior to procedure; have temporary pacer in room during procedure.
5. **Postprocedural care**
   a. Refer to Table 14.3 for neuro-interventional postprocedural care.
   b. Anticipate ICU postprocedure. Possible reperfusion injury after stent placement.
   c. May do postprocedure CT if clinical concern for hemorrhage.
   d. Resume preprocedure medications, including dual antiplatelet drugs.

6. *Follow-up*
   a. Clinic 2 weeks postprocedure.
   b. Ultrasound/duplex study within 2 weeks and 6 months postprocedure.

C. **Intracranial Angioplasty**

1. *Description*
   a. Increase caliber of narrowed intracranial vessels using a balloon (angioplasty) and/or vasodilator for arteries narrowed by vasospasm from subarachnoid hemorrhage (SAH). Arteries narrowed due to atherosclerotic plaque are dilated using balloon angioplasty with or without stent implantation to maintain vessel patency.

2. *Indications*
   a. Decrease in neurological status or delayed new focal deficit following SAH or repeated neurological events from atherosclerotic stenosis in spite of maximal medical therapy.

3. *Preprocedural work-up*
   a. Refer to Table 14.1 for neuro-interventional preprocedural care.
   b. Anticipate continued ICU postprocedure.
   c. Emergency patient's evaluation will be done in the ICU and upon arrival to the angiography suite.
   d. Have protamine, heparin, protamine, nicardipine, and abciximab available at all times.
   e. Anesthesia usually required due to pain from intracranial balloon angioplasty.

4. *Intraprocedural care*
   a. Refer to Table 14.2 for neuro-interventional intraprocedural care.
   b. Assist anesthesia if necessary; secure intracranial pressure monitor if in place.

## FAST FACTS in a NUTSHELL

- The most feared complication from intracranial angioplasty is vessel rupture.
- Always look for sudden change in vital signs or intracranial pressure, usually immediately after balloon inflation.
- Patients not under anesthesia always experience some transient discomfort during balloon inflation, but it would be more severe and persistent if the vessel ruptures.

5. *Postprocedural care*
   a. Refer to Table 14.3 for neuro-interventional postprocedural care.
   b. Continue ICU care postprocedure, possible reperfusion injury post-angioplasty.
   c. Maintain IV fluids running 0.9% NaCl.
6. *Follow-up*
   a. May do postprocedure CT if clinical concern for new hemorrhage.
   b. Patient to be followed in hospital then seen in clinic 2 weeks postprocedure or 2 weeks posthospitalization.
   c. After angioplasty for vasospasm, angiographic follow-up as per routine postaneurysm therapy, usually in 6 months, then angiography or magnetic resonance angiography annually.
   d. For angioplasty of atherosclerotic disease, angiographic or computed tomographic angiography (CTA) follow-up in 3 to 6 months and long-term follow-up with either angiography or CTA annually.
D. **Balloon Test Occlusion**
   1. *Description*
      a. Temporary occlusion of a vessel using a balloon to test for tolerance if that vessel must be occluded. Most commonly done in the internal carotid artery. The patient is tested neurologically during the test to evaluate for new neurological deficits, which would indicate that the patient would not tolerate permanent occlusion of that vessel. Often a cerebral blood flow test such as CT perfusion or nuclear medicine single photon emission computed tomography (SPECT) scans are done during the test occlusion to further evaluate what the occlusion would do to brain blood flow.
   2. *Indications*
      a. Tumor or giant aneurysm involving the vessel, which may require permanent occlusion of the vessel to treat the lesion.
   3. *Preprocedural workup*
      a. Refer to Table 14.1 for neuro-interventional preprocedural care.
      b. Coordinate with the operating room for the date and time of surgery, if planned.
      c. Coordinate the desired cerebral blood flow test that is to be done during the test.

     d. General anesthesia not usually used due to neurological testing done.

     e. Antibiotics not usually given prior to procedure.

  4. *Intraprocedural care*

     a. Refer to Table 14.2 for neuro-interventional intraprocedural care.

     b. Obtain baseline neurological status; monitor for any subtle change in neurological assessment throughout the procedure.

     c. If blood flow testing will be done, be prepared for transport to the CT scanner for CT perfusion, or have the nuclear tracer available for nuclear SPECT imaging.

     d. Document results of neurological testing.

## FAST FACTS in a NUTSHELL

- Decrease in level of consciousness or focal deficit may mean the patient cannot tolerate the occlusion.
- One trick is to give the patient a rubber squeaky toy in the hand contralateral to the vessel being occluded and have the patient squeeze it repeatedly during the balloon inflation. If the squeaking stops the patient may be developing a hemiparesis.

  5. *Postprocedural care*

     a. Refer to Table 14.3 for neuro-interventional postprocedural care.

     b. Anticipate floor status postprocedure if procedure is extracranial and no anticipation of postprocedure deficits.

     c. Head of bed elevated 20 degrees postprocedure.

  6. *Follow-up*

     a. Patient is usually seen in the clinic 2 weeks postprocedure.

     b. Imaging follow-up per surgeon.

 E. **Petrosal Venous Sampling**

  1. *Description*

     a. Patients with elevated cortisol levels may have a pituitary tumor that produces adrenocorticotropic hormone (ACTH). This is called Cushing's disease. Some of these tumors may be too small to localize on MRI scans. Sampling blood from the veins draining the pituitary may be done by catheterization and sampling from the inferior petrosal sinus. Measuring has a high accuracy of localizing the tumor in the pituitary gland, and can often determine which side of the gland is involved, allowing for surgical cure of the Cushing's disease. A stimulant of pituitary function (e.g., corticotropin-releasing hormone [CRH] or 1-deamino-8-D-arginine vasopressin [DDAVP]) is often given during the test to increase accuracy.

2. *Indications*
   a. Symptoms and laboratory evidence of Cushing's disease without a clear-cut tumor explaining the abnormal hormone production.

3. *Preprocedural workup*
   a. Refer to Table 14.1 for neuro-interventional preprocedural care.
   b. Coordinate with the lab regarding date and time of procedure. Be sure to know the proper tubes needed for the samples and make sure the lab understands the large number of samples they will be receiving and how they will be labeled.
   c. General anesthesia is not usually used due to its effect on pituitary function. Sedatives can reduce the accuracy of the test.
   d. Anticipate floor status postprocedure or may be done as outpatient.
   e. Antibiotics not usually used.
   f. Have available heparin, protamine, DDAVP, or other pituitary stimulant.
   g. Have appropriate tubes for samples, labels, worksheet to document time, site, and number of samples, and an ice bath to store the samples when transported to the lab.
   h. Ensure that each member of the team knows what his or her role will be when the samples are taken.

4. *Intraprocedural care*
   a. Refer to Table 14.2 for neuro-interventional intraprocedural care.

5. *Postprocedural care*
   a. Refer to Table 14.3 for neuro-interventional postprocedural care.
   b. Anticipate floor status postprocedure. May even be done as outpatient procedure.

- Petrosal sinus sampling requires multiple catheters with simultaneous blood samples obtained from each of the right and left petrosal sinuses and a peripheral venous sample usually obtained from a femoral venous sheath.
- These samples are obtained at various time intervals before and then repeated after the pituitary-stimulating drug (e.g., CRH or DDAVP) is given.
- Samples are tested for ACTH levels.
- Simultaneous samples mean several operators are needed to obtain the samples, then several circulators must take the samples, put them in the proper tubes, and label them carefully.
- There will be many samples with many opportunities for error.
- The results are useful only if one can be absolutely certain that the sample is correctly labeled as to whether it came from the right or left inferior petrosal sinus or peripheral vein *and* whether it was before or after pituitary stimulation.

    c. Strict bed rest with accessed legs extended for 1 hour if hemostatic patch placed or 2 to3 hours if no hemostatic agent used.

    d. Head of bed elevated 20 degrees immediately postprocedure to decrease risk of swelling.

    f. Ensure that properly labeled samples get to appropriate personnel in the lab.

6. *Follow-up*

    a. Patient will be seen in the clinic 2 weeks postprocedure.

    b. Imaging follow-up per surgeon.

- Ischemic stroke, subarachnoid hemorrhage, and other cerebrovascular conditions can be devastating for the patient but can be treated with neuro-interventional procedures.
- **Listen to your patient.** Always pay close attention to vital signs and neurological status. A sudden change can indicate something bad is happening.
- **Protect your patient.** Attention to detail with careful positioning of the patient, padding of extremities, and anticipating potential problems can keep the patient safe.
- **Talk to your patient.** Providing encouragement, support, and education can help the patient through the procedure.

# 15

# Neuro-Interventional Embolizations

## John P. Deveikis and Susan Deveikis

In this chapter, you will discover:

1. The importance of preparing for complications
2. The importance of rapid stroke care by all team members for improved outcomes
3. The nurse's role in neuro-interventional procedures

The nervous system is vitally important for normal function of the individual, yet the brain is very sensitive to ischemia. Disorders of the vascular supply to the nervous system can have devastating effects on patients and can be fatal. Neuro-interventional procedures are minimally invasive treatments for neurovascular conditions. These procedures can complement or sometimes replace more traditional medical and surgical treatments for these conditions.

# PROCEDURES

A. **Intracranial Aneurysm Embolization**
   1. *Description*
      a. Intracranial aneurysms can be treated by coil emboli-zation ("coiling"), where a small catheter (microcath-eter) is navigated through the vascular system and small, soft platinum detachable coils are delivered into the aneurysm sac to prevent blood flow into the aneurysm and thereby prevent the aneurysm from bleeding.
      b. Historically, embolization was first developed to treat patients who could not be treated with open surgical techniques (craniotomy and clipping of the aneurysm), which has been the standard treatment of aneurysms for many years. However, randomized studies have shown that outcomes of patients treated with coil em-bolization compare very favorably to those treated by open clipping. Now, increasing numbers of patients with aneurysms are treated by coiling as the primary treatment.
      c. Most of the time, the normal arteries around the aneurysm can be preserved, since the coils usually remain stable in the aneurysm sac and do not block flow in the artery. Sometimes, when there is a wide opening (neck) between the aneurysm and its parent artery, stent-assisted coiling can be done, placing a stent in the artery over the aneurysm neck to prevent the coils from protruding into the artery and possibly blocking blood flow.
      d. Some aneurysms can only be treated by blocking both the parent artery as well as the aneurysm itself, but this may impair blood flow to the brain and cause a stroke, so this is only rarely done.
      e. Recently, special stent-like devices called flow divert-ers have become available. These are deployed in the parent artery across the aneurysm neck. The stent is made of a fine meshwork of wires that can decrease flow to the aneurysm and cause it to clot off, even without the use of any coils in the aneurysm. Flow diverters such as the Pipeline embolization device (Covidien, Irvine, CA) can be used for certain

aneurysms, especially the large, wide-neck aneurysms of the carotid artery that can be difficult to treat with coil embolization.

2. *Indications*
   a. Ruptured intracranial aneurysm with subarachnoid hemorrhage (SAH).
   b. Unruptured aneurysms.
   c. Size and configuration favorable to position coils in a stable fashion.
   d. The patient should not have contraindications for arterial access (e.g., severe atherosclerotic occlusions, active bacteremia).
   e. Especially if using a stent or flow diverter, the patient should not have contraindications for use of antiplatelet medications (aspirin and clopidogrel).

3. *Preprocedural care*
   a. Refer to Table 14.1: Neuro-Interventional Preprocedural Care.
   b. Anticipate intensive care unit (ICU) stay post-procedure.
   c. Antibiotics may be given prior to implantation of coils or stents.
   d. Antiplatelet agents may be given prior to the procedure or may have been loaded several days before.
   e. Have heparin, protamine, and abciximab (ReoPro, Merck & Co., Whitehouse Station, NJ) available at all times.
   f. Evaluation per anesthesia personnel if anesthesia to be used.

## FAST FACTS in a NUTSHELL

Protamine is contraindicated in:

- Patients who are hypersensitive or intolerant to protamine.
- Insulin-dependent diabetics (may experience life-threatening anaphylaxis).
- Vasectomized males.

4. *Intraprocedural care*
   a. Refer to Table 14.2: Neuro-Interventional Preprocedural Care.

b. Ongoing neurological assessment: Anticipate worst-case scenario of aneurysm rupture, rebleed, or ischemic stroke.
c. If intracranial pressure (ICP), monitor in place. Be sure ICP monitor is clamped prior to patient transfer to angiography table. Place patient on angiography table, secure, and rezero ICP.

## FAST FACTS in a NUTSHELL

- Transducers for any pressure monitors such as arterial lines, central venous pressure, or ICP should always be attached directly to the angiography table.
- This is for safety, to prevent lines from being pulled, and for accuracy of readings.
- Remember that the angiography table may be raised and lowered multiple times during the procedure.

d. Assist anesthesia during intubation or line placement if necessary. A radial arterial line may be placed prior to induction or procedure.

## FAST FACTS in a NUTSHELL

- Always keep an eye on vital signs and the ICP monitor: A sudden change can be the first sign of aneurysm rupture.
- Any SAH patient not under anesthesia should be kept calm and in a quiet, dark, nonstimulating environment.

5. *Postprocedural care*
   a. Refer to Table 14.3: Neuro-Interventional Postprocedural Care.
   b. Anticipate bed status prior to procedure. Elective patients will need ICU bed postprocedure; ICU patient will continue in ICU postprocedure.
   c. Neurological exam upon completion of procedure and per ICU protocol, preferably every 1 hour for 24.
6. *Follow-up*
   a. If elective coiling of unruptured aneurysm, the patient may only be in the hospital for a day or two. The

patient will be seen in follow-up clinic 2 weeks post-procedure. Magnetic resonance angiography (MRA) in 6 months, 12 months, and then annually.

b. If the patient had an SAH, the patient will be seen 2 weeks after hospital discharge. SAH patients may have a prolonged hospital stay to recover from the hemorrhage. Plan arteriogram in 6 months, MRA in 12 months and then annually.

B. **Intracranial Arteriovenous Malformation (AVM) and Arteriovenous Fistula (AVF) Embolization**

1. *Description*

   a. AVM is a congenital abnormality resulting in a network (nidus) of connections between arteries and veins. AVF is a direct connection between artery and vein, which can be congenital or acquired.

2. *Indications*

   a. Rupture or risk of rupture, focal neurological symptoms, seizures, hydrocephalus, cardiac failure.

3. *Preprocedural care*

   a. Refer to Table 14.1: Neuro-Interventional Preprocedural Care.

   b. General anesthesia is usually necessary.

   c. Anticipate ICU bed postprocedure.

4. *Intraprocedural care*

   a. Refer to Table 14.2: Neuro-Interventional Intraprocedural Care.

   b. Assist anesthesia during intubation or line placement if necessary. Radial arterial line may be placed prior to induction or procedure.

5. *Postprocedural care*

   a. Refer to Table 14.3: Neuro-Interventional Postprocedural Care.

   b. Elective patients will need an ICU bed postprocedure; ICU patients will continue in ICU postprocedure.

   c. Neurological exam upon completion of procedure and per ICU protocol preferably every 1 hour × 24.

6. *Follow-up*

   a. Patient to be seen in clinic 2 weeks postprocedure or 2 weeks posthospitalization.

   b. Adults: Angiographic follow-up in 3 to 6 months.

   c. Children: Angiographic follow-up in 3 to 6 months but need long-term follow-up with either computed tomography (CT) or MRI every 2 to 3 years.

## C. Intracranial Tumor Embolization

1. *Description*
   a. Neoplastic space-occupying lesion.
2. *Indications*
   a. Reduce tumor vascularity prior to surgery.
   b. Shrink symptomatic tumors in patients who are not candidates for surgery.
3. *Preprocedural care*
   a. Refer to Table 14.1: Neuro-Interventional Preprocedural Care.
   b. Coordinate with the operating room (OR) regarding date and time of surgery. Surgery should be done within 3 to 5 days of tumor embolization.
   c. General anesthesia usually not used due to the use of provocative testing. Provocative testing is implemented to evaluate possible blood supply to nerve cell bodies or other dangerous anastomoses prior to embolization.
   d. Anticipate ICU bed postprocedure due to potential swelling of tumor postembolization.
4. *Intraprocedural care*
   a. Refer to Table 14.2: Neuro-Interventional Intraprocedural Care.
   b. For provocative testing, have methohexital sodium (Brevital, JHP Pharmaceuticals, Parsippany, NJ), lidocaine 2% cardiac bristojet, sodium bicarbonate (pediatric 0.5 mEq/mL), and 5% dextrose available.
   c. Document results of provocative testing for each vessel embolized or evaluated.

## FAST FACTS in a NUTSHELL

- Decrease in level of consciousness or severe headache may mean intracranial tumor bleeding or swelling and need for emergent intracranial surgery.
- Be prepared to obtain STAT head CT scan if bleeding is suspected.
- High-dose steroids and mannitol can sometimes control swelling prior to surgery.

5. *Postprocedural care*
    a. Refer to Table 14.3: Neuro-Interventional Postprocedural Care.
    b. Anticipate bed status prior to procedure. Elective patients will need ICU bed postprocedure; ICU patients will continue in ICU postprocedure.
    c. Head of bed elevated at least 20 degrees immediately postprocedure.
    d. Neurological exam upon completion of procedure and per ICU protocol preferably every 1 hour × 24.
6. *Follow-up*
    a. Patient will be seen in the clinic 2 weeks postprocedure.
    b. Imaging follow-up per surgeon.
D. **Extracranial Head and Neck Embolization**
    1. *Description*
        a. Block blood supply or control bleeding from a vascular lesion.
    2. *Indications*
        a. Preoperative, or to stop uncontrolled or recurrent bleeding.
    3. *Preprocedural care*
        a. Refer to Table 14.1: Neuro-Interventional Preprocedural Care.
        b. Coordinate with the OR for date and time of surgery. Surgery should ideally be done within 3 to 5 days of embolization, unless done on emergent basis.
        c. General anesthesia usually not used due to provocative testing.
        d. Anticipate floor bed after procedure; ICU usually not necessary.
    4. *Intraprocedural care*
        a. Refer to Table 14.2: Neuro-Interventional Intraprocedural Care.
        b. Point-of-care testing (activated clotting time [ACT]) capability.
        c. For provocative testing, have methohexital sodium for intra-arterial injection, lidocaine 2% cardiac bristojet, sodium bicarbonate (pediatric 0.5 mEq/mL), and 5% dextrose available.
        d. Document results of provocative testing for each vessel embolized or tested.

Preservative-free sterile water or normal saline must be used when mixing drugs for intra-arterial use.

5. *Postprocedural care*
    a. Refer to Table 14.3: Neuro-Interventional Postprocedural Care.
    b. Anticipate floor status postprocedure if procedure is extracranial and there is no anticipation of postprocedure swelling that could affect airway.
    c. Head of bed elevated 20 degrees immediately postprocedure to decrease risk of swelling.
6. *Follow-up*
    a. Patient to be seen in clinic 2 weeks postprocedure.
    b. Postimaging per surgeon.
E. **Spinal Embolization**
    1. *Description*
        a. The spine and spinal cord may be involved with vascular malformations and tumors that can be treated by catheter-based endovascular techniques. The procedure may be done prior to surgical resection of the lesion or as the primary mode of treatment. The technique is similar to what is used in the head and neck, but in the arterial supply to the spine, which often includes small branches arising directly from the aorta. Great care should be taken to avoid blocking blood flow to the spinal cord, so usually before embolizing any spinal vessel, provocative testing is done by injecting short-acting anesthetic agents (e.g., amobarbital, methohexital) into the feeding artery and testing for a transient neurological deficit. If the patient does not exhibit a new deficit, it means that the vessel to be embolized does not have any significant connection to the cord blood supply and it should be safe to embolize it.
    2. *Indications*
        a. Spinal AVF
        b. Spinal AVM
        c. Vascular tumors of the spine

3. *Preprocedural care*
   a. Refer to Table 14.1: Neuro-Interventional Preprocedural Care.
   b. Coordinate with the OR regarding date and time of surgery, if the procedure is being done preoperatively.
   c. General anesthesia not often used due to the use of provocative testing. Provocative testing is implemented to evaluate possible blood supply to nerve cell bodies or other dangerous anastomoses prior to embolization.
   d. Neurophysiological monitoring such as somatosensory-evoked potentials may or may not be used depending on physician preference and the potential risk to the spinal cord in that particular case.
   e. Anticipate ICU postprocedure if due to potential swelling postembolization.
   f. Always have heparin, protamine, dexamethasone, methohexital or amobarbital, and lidocaine on hand.
4. *Intraprocedural care*
   a. Refer to Table 14.2: Neuro-Interventional Intraprocedural Care.
   b. Conduct frequent neurological assessments and communicate any changes to attending physician immediately.
   c. Point-of-care coagulation test (ACT) capability.
5. *Postprocedural care*
   a. Refer to Table 14.3: Neuro-Interventional Postprocedural Care.
   b. Anticipate floor status postprocedure if procedure is extracranial and not directly involving spinal cord.
   c. Head of bed elevated 20 degrees immediately postprocedure for comfort.
6. *Follow-up*
   a. Patient will be seen in the clinic 2 weeks postprocedure.
   b. Imaging follow-up per surgeon.

- Ischemic stroke, SAH, and other cerebrovascular conditions can be devastating for the patient, but can be treated with neuro-interventional procedures.
- **Listen to your patient.** Always pay close attention to vital signs and neurological status. A sudden change can indicate something bad is happening.
- **Protect your patient.** Attention to detail with careful positioning of the patient, padding of extremities, and anticipating potential problems can keep the patient safe.
- **Talk to your patient.** Providing encouragement, support, and education can help the patient through the procedure.

# 16

# Basic (Body) Interventional Radiology Principles

## Ayman Sawas and Ashwani Kumar Sharma

In this chapter, you will discover:

1. The importance of aseptic technique
2. Procedural antibiotic use
3. Key lab values

## STERILE FIELD AND ASEPTIC TECHNIQUE

Sterile technique is aimed at reducing the rate of infections of wounds and implanted devices, which is very important in the context of procedures in interventional radiology (IR). Bacteria colonize on the skin, on equipment, and in the air of the angiographic suite. To protect the patient and staff:

- Proper hand scrubbing *must* be performed with soap and water or an alcohol-based skin rub and hands *must* be thoroughly dried.
- Disposable gown, head cap, mask, and gloves must be worn for each procedure.
- Double gloving can reduce the risk of perforation and cross infection.

- Care must be taken to drape the patient as well as the image intensifier and the ultrasound prop if they are going to be used in a procedure.
- The procedure site should be prepped in aseptic technique.
- Patient's hair should be clipped at the site of the procedure and the skin should be vigorously scrubbed with 2% chlorhexidine-based preparation for 2 minutes. Alternatively, povidone–iodine can be used if the patient has an allergy to chlorhexidine. Allow to dry per manufacturer's recommendations prior to draping patient.
- All sterile packages used for the procedure should be checked for package integrity and expiration dates when applicable.

## *FAST FACTS in a NUTSHELL*

Sterile technique is crucial for reducing the rate of infections in all IR procedures as well as improving patient care. Further information on sterile technique can be found on the U.S. Department of Health and Human Services website at the following link: www.guideline.gov/content.aspx?id=12921#Section420.

## ANTIBIOTICS

Prophylactic antibiotics can be given with some IR procedures to reduce the chance of surgical site infection and seeding of foreign bodies. The careful timing of intravenous (IV) antimicrobial prophylaxis should be one of the following:

- Administered within 1 hour before and up to 3 hours after the intervention.
- Two hours prior to intervention are allowed for the administration of vancomycin and fluoroquinolones.
- IV antibiotics are usually given when the patient arrives to the angiography suite.
- The choice of antibiotic depends on the procedure.
  - In **clean vascular procedures** such as central venous catheter placement, a first-generation cephalosporin such as 1 g of cefazolin IV is usually used; alternatively, vancomycin can be used in patients with a penicillin or cephalosporin allergy.

## TABLE 16.1 Prophylactic Procedural Antibiotic Recommendations

| Procedures | Routine Prophylaxis Recommendation | First Choice of Antibiotics | Alternative Antibiotics for Patients With Penicillin Allergy |
|---|---|---|---|
| Angiography, angioplasty, thrombolysis, arterial closure device placement, stent placement | No | Cefazolin in patients with risk for stent infection | Vancomycin or clindamycin |
| Biliary/liver procedures | Yes | No consensus. Some may use ceftriaxone, Unasyn, or Zosyn | Vancomycin or clindamycin |
| Embolization and chemoembolization | Yes | No consensus. Some may use ceftriaxone, cefazolin and metronidazole, Unasyn, or Zosyn | Vancomycin |
| Gastrostomy | Yes for pull technique | Cefazolin | Vancomycin or clindamycin |
| Genitourinary procedures (include nephrostomy tubes and ureteral stents) | Yes (except for routine change in uninfected patients) | No consensus. Some may use ceftriaxone, cefazolin, Unasyn, or ampicillin and gentamicin. | Vancomycin or clindamycin and aminoglycoside |
| Percutaneous abscess drainage | Yes | No consensus. Some may use ceftriaxone, cefoxitin, cefotetan, or Unasyn | Vancomycin or clindamycin or aminoglycoside |
| Percutaneous biopsy (nontransrectal) | No | None | None |
| Percutaneous biopsy (transrectal) | Yes | Gentamicin plus ciprofloxacin | |
| Transjugular intrahepatic portosystemic shunt (TIPSS) creation | Yes | No consensus. Some may use ceftriaxone, Unasyn, or Zosyn | Vancomycin or clindamycin and aminoglycoside |
| Tunneled central venous access | No consensus | Cefazolin in patients with history of catheter infection or immunosuppression | Vancomycin or clindamycin |
| Tumor ablation | No consensus | Some may use ceftriaxone, cefazolin, or Unasyn | Vancomycin or clindamycin |
| Uterine artery embolization | Yes | No consensus. Some may use cefazolin, clindamycin and gentamycin, or Unasyn | Vancomycin or clindamycin |
| Vertebroplasty | Yes | Cefazolin | Vancomycin or clindamycin |

*Source:* Bratzler et al. (2013); Cunha (2013); Venkatesan et al. (2010).

- **Gram-negative bacterial** coverage in urinary procedures such as **nephrostomy** tube placement is desired, and ciprofloxacin 400 mg IV can provide adequate prophylaxis.
- **Biliary interventions** such as a percutaneous biliary drain require both gram-positive and gram-negative bacterial coverage and an antibiotic with extended coverage such as Zosyn.
- Some of these antibiotics may require dose adjustment in patients with renal insufficiency.
- Refer to Table 16.1 for prophylactic procedural antibiotic guidelines during IR procedures.

## COAGULATION STATUS AND HOMEOSTASIS

Procedures performed in IR sometimes entail puncturing of blood vessels or cause damage to vascular organs such as the kidney or liver. Therefore, these procedures usually carry the risk of bleeding or developing a hematoma. It is important to screen patients for bleeding risk and to maintain homeostasis during the procedure.

### *FAST FACTS in a NUTSHELL*

In emergent situations or in certain cases, an interventional procedure can be performed if the benefits of the procedure outweigh the bleeding risk.

Several tests are used to assess the bleeding risk in patients; these include:

- Prothrombin time (PT)
  - Measure the extrinsic coagulation pathway
  - Value can vary depending on assay used in particular lab
- International normalized ratio (INR)
  - Measure of the extrinsic coagulation pathway
  - Result is standardized and more dependable
  - Normal range is 0.9 to 1.1
- Activated partial thromboplastin time (aPTT)
  - Measure of the intrinsic coagulation pathway
  - Normal range for aPTT is 25 to 35 seconds
  - Patients receiving heparin or who have hemophilia may have an aPTT value of more than 50 seconds

- Platelet count
  - Normal platelet count is 150,000 to 450,000/mcL
    - ⇒ Liver disease, vitamin deficiency, and oral anticoagulation therapy such as Coumadin (warfarin) can impair coagulation, resulting in a prolonged PT and elevated INR.
    - ⇒ The target for patients on Coumadin therapy is usually an INR of 2 to 3.5.
    - ⇒ Patients on anticoagulation therapy or who may have liver disease should have an INR/PT check prior to IR procedures.
    - ⇒ Patients on heparin drips should have heparin drip discontinued 1 to 2 hours prior to the procedure or an aPTT can be checked.

*The Journal of Vascular and Interventional Radiology* consensus guidelines divide the procedure into different categories depending on the risk of bleeding associated with the procedure.

- Category 1 is low-bleeding-risk procedures such as venography, inferior vena cava (IVC), filter placement, peripherally inserted central catheter (PICC) placement, central line removal, drainage catheter exchange, and thoracentesis.
  - No routine testing of platelets or INR is recommended for these low-risk procedures; for patients with risk factors, the INR should be less than 2.0 and platelets should be more than 50,000/mcL.
- Category 2 is moderate bleeding risk procedures such as angiography, venous interventions, tunneled central venous catheter insertion, chemoembolization, transjugular liver biopsy, lung biopsy, nephrostomy tube, radiofrequency ablation, and lung biopsy.
  - Routine testing for INR is recommended, but no routine testing of platelets is recommended for these moderate risk procedures.
  - In patients with risk factors, the INR should be less than 1.5 and platelets should be more than 50,000/mcL.
- Category 3 is significant bleeding risk procedures such as transjugular intrahepatic portosystemic shunt (TIPSS), renal biopsy, biliary interventions, and nephrostomy tube placement.
  - Routine testing of platelets and INR is recommended for these high-risk procedures.
  - The INR should be less than 1.5 and platelets should be more than 50,000 per mcL.

See Table 16.2, Coagulation Evaluation for Interventional Procedures.

## TABLE 16.2 Coagulation Evaluation for Interventional Procedures

| Bleeding Risk | Procedure | Recommendations |
|---|---|---|
| Category 1: Low risk for bleeding | Dialysis access interventions<br>Venography<br>Central line removal<br>IVC filter placement<br>PICC placement<br>Drainage catheter exchange<br>Thoracentesis<br>Paracentesis<br>Superficial aspiration<br>Superficial soft tissue biopsy (ex-thyroid biopsy)<br>Superficial abscess drainage | Lab screening for patients with risk factors:<br>INR < 2<br>Platelets > 50,000/mcL<br>Plavix: hold for 5 days |
| Category 2: Moderate risk for bleeding | Angiography<br>Venous interventions<br>Tunneled central venous catheter<br>Subcutaneous port device<br>Uterine fibroid embolization<br>Chemoembolization/radioembolization<br>Radiofrequency ablation<br>Percutaneous cholecystostomy<br>Intra-abdominal, chest wall, or retroperitoneal abscess drainage or biopsy<br>Lung biopsy<br>Liver biopsy<br>Gastrostomy tube initial placement<br>Spine procedures (vertebroplasty, kyphoplasty) | Routine INR screening. Platelet and aPTT screening in patients with risk factors:<br>INR < 1.5<br>Platelets > 50,000/mcL<br>Plavix: hold for 5 days |
| Category 3: High risk for bleeding | Transjugular intrahepatic portosystemic shunt (TIPSS)<br>Renal biopsy<br>PTC (percutaneous transhepatic cholangiogram)<br>Biliary drain initial placement<br>Nephrostomy tube initial placement<br>Radiofrequency ablation | Routine INR and platelet screening. aPTT screening in patients with risk factors.<br>INR < 1.5<br>Platelets > 50,000/mcL<br>Plavix: hold for 5 days<br>Aspirin: hold for 5 days |

Source: Patel et al. (2012).

**Plavix** (clopidogrel) should be held for 5 days prior to any IR procedure. This sometimes requires consultation with the patient's cardiologist to ensure patient safety while Plavix is held. **Aspirin** should be held for 5 days prior to procedures with significant bleeding risks. Routine withholding is not recommended for low and moderate bleeding risk procedures. **Low molecular weight heparin** or **Lovenox** therapeutic doses should be held for 24 hours prior to the procedure, while IV heparin drip should be held for 2 hours prior to the procedure, as heparin has a half-life of approximately 1.5 hours.

Correction of coagulopathy may be necessary in patients requiring a procedure when the INR level or platelet counts do not meet the required recommendations.

- Fresh frozen plasma (FFP) contains plasma proteins, including coagulation factors, and can be administered to patients with an elevated INR.

═══════════════════════════════════*FAST FACTS in a NUTSHELL*

Two units of FFP are usually sufficient to correct an INR of 2.5.

- When a procedure is emergently required for a patient with an elevated aPTT from a heparin drip and the procedure cannot be delayed, reversal medication (protamine sulfate) can be administered. Protamine dose is 1 mg per 100 units of heparin and has a rapid onset in 10 minutes; however, it has a short half-life of 5 to 7.5 minutes and repeat administration of protamine can be necessary.
- Patients with thrombocytopenia below the recommended platelet counts should receive platelet transfusion prior to the procedure. Four to six units of random platelets or one unit of pooled platelets are usually given and raise the platelet count by an estimated 30,000/mcL.

## MANAGEMENT OF CRITICALLY ILL PATIENTS

Patients who are critically ill are sometimes referred to IR for life-saving treatment. It is imperative for IR staff to be familiar with the basics of assessment and life support management. Such cases include patients suffering from traumatic injury, patients with hemorrhage, and severe disease such as liver failure or sepsis. Monitoring of these patients to identify life-threatening problems during a procedure must be routinely performed. Nurses should observe the breathing rate and oxygen saturation during the procedure and alert the physician for abnormal values. **Hypoxia** and hypoventilation during a procedure can be caused by many different reasons, including pneumothorax due to traumatic or iatrogenic injury, lung collapse due to mucous plugging, pulmonary edema or pleural effusion due to underlying systemic disease, and decreased respiratory drive due to sedation. When patients are hypoxic (pulse oximetry of less than 88% to 92%) the staff should consider applying or increasing supplemental oxygen with nasal cannula or a high-flow oxygen mask, identifying and treating the underlying cause. Intubation may be required if the patient is in respiratory failure.

**Circulatory compromise** during a procedure can be caused by many different reasons, including hemorrhage due to traumatic injury or gastrointestinal bleeding. It is important to recognize that patients with:

- Hemorrhagic Class 1 hemorrhage, which is classified as up to 15% loss of blood volume, but with no significant change in vital signs.
- Hemorrhagic Class 2 hemorrhage, which is classified as a blood loss of up to 30% of blood volume and the early significant change is manifested by tachycardia and tachypnea.
- Hemorrhagic Class 3 hemorrhage, which is classified as 30% to 40% blood volume loss, results in oliguria, restlessness, and changed in skin perfusion.
- Hemorrhagic Class 4 hemorrhage, which is classified as > 40% blood volume loss, results in hypotension, heart rate > 140 bpm and lethargy.
  - Adequate volume resuscitation is necessary when patients have signs of volume loss.
  - Initial volume resuscitation is initiated with crystalloid IV fluids such as normal saline or lactated Ringer's solution.
  - Patients with hemorrhage may remain hypovolemic and after 1 to 2 L of crystalloid IV fluid may require packed red blood cell (PRBC) transfusions.
  - After 4 to 6 units of PRBC are transfused, other blood products such as FFP, platelet, and cryoprecipitate can be considered (Glorsky, Wonderlich, & Gori, 2010).

Patients with a left ventricular assist device (LVAD) may have a lower baseline automated blood pressure cuff measurement than non-LVAD patients. It could be as low as a systolic of 90 mmHg and be considered normal for that patient (Myers, Bolmers, Gregoric, Kar, & Frazier, 2009).

## ANESTHESIA

Interventional procedures can be uncomfortable to patients and can cause significant anxiety; therefore, medications are often used with these procedures to make patients more comfortable. Available options for analgesia and anesthesia include local anesthesia, local anesthesia with sedation, regional anesthesia, and general anesthesia. Local anesthesia with moderate sedation is often employed in IR procedures.

- Infiltration of the skin with lidocaine 1% is used for local anesthesia. If a patient has an allergy to lidocaine, then procaine (Novocain) can be used.
- Moderate sedation can be achieved by administering a combination of benzodiazepine and opioid medications (refer to Chapter 6 for more information).
- Reversal agents include flumazenil and naloxone, and should be readily available.
- Patient should be given nothing by mouth (NPO) prior to the procedure, per institution policy. Usually no food or non-clear liquids for 6 to 8 hours and no clear liquids for 2 hours prior to administration of moderate sedation.
- Blood pressure, electrocardiogram (ECG), pulse oximetry, respiratory rate, and temperature should be monitored during procedures with sedation; vital signs should be recorded every 5 to 15 minutes per organization policy. Supplemental oxygen with nasal cannula can be utilized to maintain the patient's oxygenation.
- Postprocedural monitoring of patients for 30 minutes after the administration of the last dose of sedation is required.
- Some procedures can be performed with minimal sedation and only local anesthesia utilizing 1% lidocaine. Intraoperative

monitoring for these procedures is limited to blood pressure and ECG monitoring.

General anesthesia performed by the anesthesia service is indicated in cases when it is difficult to maintain a patient's airway with sedation, muscle relaxation is needed, or when patients desire a higher level of anesthesia. In pediatric cases, a pediatric specialist or anesthesia services are usually utilized for sedation.

Tables 16.3 to 16.5 refer to care routine for most IR procedures.

### TABLE 16.3 Preprocedural Care

1. Nothing by mouth after midnight.
2. Identification/consideration of pregnant/nonpregnant state.
3. Remove all jewelry and secure per organizational policy.
4. Have patient void.
5. For outpatients, designated driver should be present prior to procedure.
6. Verify medical history including allergies and pregnancy, perform physical assessment including vital signs, and ensure appropriate lab results are up to date.
7. Consent forms signed (procedural, sedation, blood, do not resuscitate [DNR] order, and so on).
8. Baseline vital signs (including lung sounds, pedal pulses, and so on, as appropriate).
9. Peripheral IV line(s).
10. Anticipate postprocedure bed status.
11. Check distal pulses before and after angiograms.

## TABLE 16.4 Intraprocedural Care

1. Verify patient identification upon arrival to angiography suite.
2. Check with operator for patient positioning.
3. Never leave patient unattended. Provide emotional support to patient.
4. Place patient on hemodynamic monitors (ECG, heart rate, blood pressure, respiratory rate, and oxygen saturation) and obtain baseline vital signs.
5. Monitor and record throughout procedure per organization policy.
6. Ultrasound, fluoroscopy, or CT may be used depending on the case.
7. Access site as determined by the physician.
8. Hair at the site should be clipped and the residue should be removed with tape (when appropriate).
9. Prep and drape in a sterile manner (follow manufacturer's recommendations for drying time of skin prep prior to draping patient).
10. "Time out" and procedural verification prior to start of procedure, per organization policy.
11. Samples obtained during a procedure require adequate labeling and handling per organization policy.

## TABLE 16.5 Postprocedural Care

1. Monitor patients in the postprocedure recovery area per organizational policy.
2. Check access/puncture site for bleeding upon completion of the procedure, then hourly for signs of complications.
3. Check distal pulses before and after angiograms.
4. Resume preprocedure diet and medications as indicated.
5. For outpatients, discharge instructions with contact information should be provided. Advise patient to seek medical attention if having swelling at procedure site, fevers, chills, or signs of allergic reaction.

# 17

# Interventions for Varicose Veins

**Ayman Sawas and Ashwani Kumar Sharma**

In this chapter, you will discover:

1. A description of varicose veins
2. The different treatments available for varicose veins
3. An understanding of necessary patient care

Varicose veins are dilated, tortuous, and elongated veins that can affect both males and females. Some studies suggest prevalence of up to 56% in men and 73% in women. Patients with varicose veins can complain of cosmetic deformity, pruritus, pain, swelling, cramping, or heaviness. A few patients may develop complications of varicose veins including thrombophlebitis, varicose eczema, lipodermatosclerosis, ulceration, and venous thrombosis.

The veins of the lower extremity are divided into three categories—superficial, perforating, and deep veins. Superficial veins drain blood from the skin and subcutaneous tissues, act as a large reservoir, and drain periodically into larger superficial veins or into the deep venous system via the perforating veins. Normally, flow should be in the cephalad direction and drain from the superficial to deep venous system. The deep veins are located deep to the muscle fascia in the legs and drain blood from muscles and blood that they receive from the superficial venous system via the perforating veins. The greater saphenous vein (GSV) is the largest of the superficial veins. The lesser saphenous vein (LSV) is the second truncal superficial vein.

Imaging studies are not generally necessary for diagnosis but are important for workup prior to planning treatment procedures. Evaluation of varicose veins is primarily evaluated by duplex ultrasound examination.

## FAST FACTS in a NUTSHELL

The physical examination for the superficial veins is performed with the patient standing, as that increases sensitivity and specificity.

## ABLATION FOR VARICOSE VEINS

A. **Introduction**
  1. Endovenous laser ablation (EVLA) and radiofrequency ablation (RFA) are treatments for varicose veins because of reflux in the GSV and LSV. These work by inducing a thermal injury to the vein, which causes eventual fibrosis of the vein.
  2. Puncture is made into the vein of interest and a vascular sheath is advanced into the vein. A laser sheet with catheter or radiofrequency probe is then positioned appropriately under ultrasound or fluoroscopic guidance to perform the ablation.
B. **Indications**
  1. Symptomatic varicose veins with reflux in the GSV or LSV and nonsaphenous veins.
  2. Venous ulcers.
  3. Varicose vein bleeding.
C. **Contraindications**
  1. Deep venous thrombosis (DVT).
  2. Pregnancy.
  3. Moderate to severe peripheral disease.
  4. Joint disease that interferes with mobility.
D. **Preprocedural care workup**
  1. Refer to Table 16.3 for preprocedural care.
E. **Anesthesia**
  1. Procedure usually performed with perivenous tumescent anesthesia. Perivenous tumescent anesthesia is achieved by injecting local anesthetic such as lidocaine around the

vein targeted for therapy. Moderate sedation can also be given depending on the patient.

F. **Intraprocedural care**
   1. Refer to Table 16.4 for intraprocedural care.
   2. Patient placed on fluoroscopy table, usually in supine position for greater saphenous vein and prone for LSV ablation.
   3. The procedure is performed with ultrasound and/or fluoroscopy.

G. **Postprocedural care**
   1. Refer to Table 16.5 for postprocedural care.
   2. Check site for bleeding or hematoma.
   3. Pain control with acetaminophen or codeine. Nonsteroidal anti-inflammatory drugs (NSAIDs) should be **avoided**, as these medications inhibit the inflammatory process, which is part of the goal of therapy to treat the varicose veins.

H. **Follow-up/patient education**
   1. Follow-up with interventional radiology 1 week postprocedure.
   2. Patient should ambulate for 15 to 20 minutes several times a day.
   3. Compression stockings should be worn for 1 to 3 weeks postprocedure. Patient may develop numbness in the lower extremities due to compression stockings; this can require removal of stockings and/or using lower-pressure stockings.
   4. Avoid heavy lifting and strenuous activities for 1 to 2 weeks. Patient can usually return to normal activities in 3 to 7 weeks.
   5. Ultrasound to evaluate for DVT in 1 week. The most concerning complication following EVLA therapy is the development of a DVT, occurring in up to 5% of patients. It is for this reason that a follow-up ultrasound examination is performed approximately 1 week after the procedure.
   6. Other possible complications include skin burn, nerve injury, and superficial thrombophlebitis. Superficial thrombophlebitis is a complication that is self-limited, peaks at 4 to 7 days, and resolves in approximately a week. Treatment includes ice packing. NSAIDs should be avoided but can be used.

7. Discharge instructions should advise the patient to seek medical attention if there is swelling at the puncture site, swelling of the extremity, or severe pain suggesting DVT.

# PHLEBECTOMY FOR VARICOSE VEINS

A. **Introduction**
   1. Phlebectomy is an ambulatory procedure that involves removal of varicose veins.
   2. Skin incisions as small as 1 to 3 mm or needle punctures are used to extract veins with a phlebectomy hook.
B. **Indications**
   1. Symptomatic varicose veins that are tortuous.
   2. The same indication for ablation but in cases that cannot be treated by ablation.
C. **Contraindications**
   1. Reflux at the saphenofemoral or saphenopopliteal junctions, which should be treated first, before phlebectomy.
D. **Preprocedural care**
   1. Refer to Table 16.3 for preprocedural care.
E. **Anesthesia**
   2. Procedure usually performed with perivenous tumescent anesthesia.
F. **Intraprocedural care**
   1. Refer to Table 16.4 for intraprocedural care.
   2. Patient placed on fluoroscopy table, usually in supine position.
   3. Ultrasound or vein light usually used.
   4. After allowing for drainage of anesthesia fluid, large pads are applied along the site of vein removal and covered with an inelastic bandage.
   5. An elastic bandage or compression stockings are then applied.
G. **Postprocedural care**
   1. Refer to Table 16.5 for postprocedural care.
   2. If patient is having bleeding, then gentle pressure is applied. Leg elevation for 5 to 10 minutes postprocedure can be useful.
   3. Pain control.
H. **Follow-up/patient education**
   1. Follow-up with interventional radiology 4 to 6 weeks postprocedure.

2. Patient should ambulate for 15 to 20 minutes several times a day.
3. Dressings can be removed in 1 to 2 days.
4. Compression stockings should be worn for 1 to 3 weeks postprocedure. Patient may develop numbness in the lower extremities due to compression stockings. This can require removal of stockings and using lower-pressure stockings.
5. Avoid heavy lifting and strenuous activities for 1 to 2 weeks. Patient can usually return to normal activities in 3 to 7 days.
6. Ultrasound to evaluate for DVT is performed initially to exclude the presence of a rare complication. Ultrasound follow-up in 1 to 4 weeks after treatment is recommended by the Union Internationale de Phlebologie to determine the success of therapy and to evaluate for recurrence of varicose veins.
7. Bruising and hyperpigmentation usually resolve in several months.
8. Follow-up with interventional radiology in 4 to 6 weeks postprocedure.
9. Other complications include pain, varicose vein recurrence, edema, bruising bleeding, hyperpigmentation, tissue necrosis, thrombophlebitis, DVT, telangiectasia, and sensory deficits.
10. Discharge instructions should advise patient to seek medical attention if there is swelling at the puncture site or of the extremity suggesting DVT.

## VENOGRAPHY

A. **Description**
   1. Venography is a procedure used for assessing the anatomy and flow in veins.
   2. Access is obtained distal or upstream to the region of interest and contrast agent injected under fluoroscopy to visualize the region of interest.
B. **Indications**
   1. Evaluation for DVT.
   2. Venous malformation.
   3. Evaluation for tumor encasement of venous structures.
   4. Evaluation for fistula creation.

C. **Contraindications**
   1. Pregnancy.
D. **Preprocedural care**
   1. Refer to Table 16.3 for preprocedural care.
E. **Anesthesia**
   1. Procedure is usually performed with local anesthesia and minimal sedation.
   2. Moderate sedation can also be used.
F. **Intraprocedural care**
   1. Refer to Table 16.4 for intraprocedural care.
   2. Patient placed on fluoroscopy table, usually in supine position.
   3. Ultrasound maybe used for identifying the venous site initially and then fluoroscopy.
   4. For DVT, dorsum veins of the foot are used for access and injection.
   5. Tourniquet or blood pressure cuff can be utilized to prevent filling of superficial veins.
G. **Postprocedural care**
   1. Refer to Table 16.5 for postprocedural care.
   2. Complications of the procedure include entry site hematoma, contrast extravasation into subcutaneous soft tissue, contrast-induced nephropathy, contrast reaction, infection, and thrombophlebitis.
   3. Refer to Chapter 10 for the treatment of contrast reactions.
H. **Follow-up/patient education**
   1. Outpatient follow-up in 4 to 6 weeks.

## *FAST FACTS in a NUTSHELL*

- The goal of ablation and sclerotherapy is to cause fibrosis of the varicose vein. NSAIDs can interfere with this process and, therefore, should be avoided.
- Patients are at risk of developing DVT after the procedure. An ultrasound to evaluate for DVT is usually performed within the first week after the procedure.

## SCLEROTHERAPY

A. **Introduction**
   1. Sclerotherapy is an alternative treatment for varicose veins.

2. A sclerosing agent is injected into the abnormal veins while avoiding damage to other vessels. This agent causes endothelial and vessel wall damage, resulting in obliteration of the vein into a thread of connective tissue.
3. Ultrasound can be employed in this procedure to visualize and access the abnormal veins.

B. **Indications**
1. Symptomatic small varicose veins.
2. Spider veins.
3. Remnant veins after ablative therapy and phlebectomy.
4. Cosmetic purposes.

C. **Contraindications**
1. Allergy to sclerosing agents.
2. Veins thrombosis or acute thrombophlebitis.
3. Hypercoagulable state.
4. Peripheral vascular disease.
5. Patent foramen ovale.
6. Immobility.
7. Pregnancy.

D. **Preprocedural care**
1. Refer to Table 16.3 for preprocedural care.

E. **Anesthesia**
1. Procedure is usually performed with perivenous tumescent anesthesia.

F. **Intraprocedural care**
1. Refer to Table 16.4 for intraprocedural care.
2. Positioning of the patient depends on site of sclerotherapy.
3. Ultrasound can be used to access the veins.

G. **Postprocedural care**
1. Refer to Table 16.5 for postprocedural care.
2. Pain control with acetaminophen or codeine. NSAIDs should be avoided because these medications inhibit the inflammatory process, which is part of the goal of therapy to treat the varicose veins.

H. **Follow-up/patient education**
1. Patient should ambulate for 15 to 20 minutes several times a day.
2. Compression stockings should be worn for 1 to 3 weeks postprocedure.
3. Avoid heavy lifting and strenuous activities for 1 to 2 weeks. Patient can usually return to normal activities in 3 to 7 days.
4. Ultrasound to evaluate for DVT is performed in 1 week.

5. Follow-up with interventional radiology 4 to 6 weeks postprocedure.
6. Other complications include anaphylaxis, pain, bruising, hyperpigmentation, tissue necrosis, thrombophlebitis, DVT, stroke, visual changes, and cough.

# 18

# Central Venous Catheters

## Ayman Sawas and Ashwani Kumar Sharma

In this chapter, you will discover:

1. The purpose of placing a central venous catheter
2. The importance of ECG monitoring during the procedure
3. How to care for the central venous catheter

## CENTRAL VENOUS CATHETERS

A. **Introduction**
   1. Central venous catheters are placed to allow access to the large veins.
   2. These catheters can be used for therapeutic treatment and diagnostic evaluation.
   3. Catheters used in this procedure vary in size, number of lumens, sites of insertion, and duration of use. They include tunneled central venous catheters, dialysis catheters, plasmapheresis catheters, nontunneled venous catheters, and peripherally inserted venous catheters.

4. Use of image guidance by interventional radiology allows for a faster and safer insertion of such catheters.

5. Access to the large vein, such as the internal jugular vein, is gained using ultrasound; fluoroscopy is then used to complete the procedure.

B. **Indications**

1. Administration of intravenous (IV) fluids and medications including those that may not be administered peripherally such as vasopressors, chemotherapeutic drugs and antibiotics, blood products transfusion, and total parental nutrition.

2. Plasmapheresis.

3. Hemodialysis.

4. Hemodynamic monitoring.

5. Poor peripheral venous access.

6. Repeated blood sampling.

C. **Contraindications**

1. Cellulitis at the site of insertion.

2. Bacteremia.

3. Venous collusion of the veins chosen for insertion.

4. Coagulopathy.

D. **Preprocedural care**

1. Refer to Table 16.3 for preprocedural care.

E. **Anesthesia**

1. Procedure usually performed with moderate sedation and local anesthesia.

F. **Intraprocedural care**

1. Refer to Table 16.4 for intraprocedural care.

2. Patient placed on fluoroscopy table, usually in supine position.

3. Site is evaluated with ultrasound to evaluate for patency. The right internal jugular vein is usually preferred for access, followed by the left side subclavian veins and femoral veins, respectively. Fluoroscopy may then be used.

4. Prophylactic antibiotics should be given if the patient is not receiving IV antibiotics, usually first-generation cephalosporin such as cefazolin IV. Alternatives include vancomycin.

5. A protective skin disk such as chlorhexidine disk and clear sterile occlusive dressing are applied to the catheter site. There are usually two skin incisions made for tunneled catheter central lines; the internal jugular venous

site should be dressed with gauze and clear occlusive dressing.

6. The catheter ports are flushed with normal saline to clear them of blood.

7. Catheters are usually locked with heparin depending on the type of catheter. If the patient is allergic to heparin, then tissue plasminogen activator can be used.

## FAST FACTS in a NUTSHELL

Special attention should be paid to electrocardiogram (ECG) monitoring when catheters are placed within the cardiac chambers due to possibility of arrhythmia.

G. **Postprocedural care**
  1. Refer to Table 16.5 for basic postprocedural care.
  2. Assess for shortness of breath, as this can be a sign of pneumothorax.
  3. Postprocedural chest x-ray is routinely performed to evaluate for pneumothorax, other complications related to the procedure, and positioning of the catheter.
  4. Complications of the procedure include bleeding, infection, and injury to the surrounding structures at the insertion site such as nerves, arterial placement, or pneumothorax.

H. **Follow-up/patient education**
  1. Catheters require routine dressing changes.
  2. Catheters should be routinely flushed after cleaning the port hub.
  3. Catheters should be removed when they are no longer needed. This can be done at bedside or as an outpatient with or without minimal sedation.

## TOTALLY IMPLANTABLE VENOUS ACCESS SYSTEM (PORT-A-CATH, MEDIPORT)

A. **Introduction**
  1. Totally implantable venous access systems are a special type of central venous catheter, with all components placed under the skin.

2. These are commonly used for chemotherapy drug injections.
3. These catheters have a palpable reservoir component where a needle can be inserted through the skin for accessing the port.
4. A skin incision at the upper chest that is several centimeters in length is made during the procedure for initial placement of the reservoir component.
5. Access to the large vein, such as the internal jugular vein, is gained using ultrasound, then fluoroscopy is used to complete the procedure.

B. **Indications**
   1. Administration of chemotherapeutic drugs.

C. **Contraindications**
   1. Cellulites at the site of insertion.
   2. Bacteremia.
   3. Venous collusion of the veins chosen for insertion.
   4. Coagulopathy.

D. **Preprocedural care**
   1. Refer to Table 16.3 for preprocedural care.

E. **Anesthesia**
   1. Procedure usually performed with moderate sedation and local anesthesia.

F. **Intraprocedural care**
   1. Refer to Table 16.4 for intraprocedural care.
   2. Patient placed on fluoroscopy table, usually in supine position.
   3. Special attention should be paid to ECG monitoring when catheters are placed within the cardiac chambers due to the possibility of arrhythmia.
   4. Ultrasound is used to evaluate for patency. The right internal jugular vein is usually preferred for access, followed by the left side subclavian and femoral veins, respectively. Fluoroscopy will then be used.
   5. Prophylactic antibiotics should be given if the patient is not receiving intravenous (IV) antibiotics, usually first-generation cephalosporin such as cefazolin IV. Alternatives include vancomycin.
   6. Protective skin dressing or Steri-Strips are applied to close the skin incisions.
   7. The catheter port is flushed with normal saline and locked with heparin per manufacturer and organization policy.

G. **Postprocedural care**
1. Refer to Table 16.5 for postprocedural care.
2. Assess for shortness of breath, as this can be a sign of pneumothorax.
3. Postprocedural chest x-ray is routinely performed to evaluate for pneumothorax, other complications related to the procedure, and positioning of the catheter.
4. Complications of the procedure include bleeding, infection, and injury to the surrounding structures at the insertion site such as nerves, arterial placement, or pneumothorax.

H. **Follow-up/patient education**
1. Routine outpatient follow-up in 1 week to assess the port site. The port can be accessed during this period if needed.
2. Catheters should be removed when they are no longer needed. Removal requires an outpatient procedure with moderate sedation to remove all port components.

# 19

## Dialysis Access

**Ayman Sawas and Ashwani Kumar Sharma**

In this chapter, you will discover:

1. The stages of chronic kidney disease
2. The importance of pulse assessments pre- and postprocedure
3. Procedural complications

## PROCEDURAL CARE FOR PATIENTS WITH CHRONIC KIDNEY DISEASE

Chronic renal disease is a worldwide health problem, with rising incidence and prevalence resulting in poor outcomes and high cost. In 2000, the National Kidney Foundation (NKF) Kidney Disease Outcome Quality Initiative (KDOQI) Advisory Board approved development of clinical practice guidelines to define chronic kidney disease and to classify stages in the progression of chronic kidney disease. The work group charged with developing the guidelines consisted of experts in nephrology, pediatric nephrology, epidemiology, laboratory medicine, nutrition, social work, gerontology, and family medicine. The definition of chronic renal disease as defined by the KDOQI work group is as follows:

1. Kidney damage for up to 3 months, as defined by structural or functional abnormalities of the kidney, with or without decreased glomerular filtration rate (eGFR), manifest by *either:*
   - Pathologic abnormalities
   - Markers of kidney damage, including abnormalities in the composition of the blood or urine, or abnormalities in imaging tests
2. eGFR less than 60 mL/min/1.73 $m^2$ for up to 3 months, with or without kidney damage

## *FAST FACTS in a NUTSHELL*

- Check and document pulses of the major arteries in the arm before and after the procedure.
- Heparin is given during the procedure to prevent fistula thrombosis.
- The patient may require dialysis after the procedure depending on labs and fluid status.

**Chronic Kidney Disease Classification:**
- Stage 1: eGFR of 90 mL/min/1.73 $m^2$ or greater
  - Diagnosis and treatment of the primary disease
- Stage 2: eGFR of 60 to 89 mL/min/1.73 $m^2$
  - Monitoring the disease
- Stage 3: eGFR of 30 to 59 mL/min/1.73 $m^2$
  - Primary disease complication management
- Stage 4: eGFR of 15 to 29 mL/min/1.73 $m^2$
  - Getting ready for kidney replacement therapy
- Stage 5: eGFR less than 15 mL/min/1.73 $m^2$
  - Dialysis and/or renal replacement

According to the NKF KDOQI guidelines, tunneled cuffed venous catheters are indicated for temporary venous access that is expected to be required for longer than 3 weeks and may serve as a bridging device during maturation of newly placed arteriovenous fistulas (AVFs) or as the final option for patients in whom fistulas and grafts have failed.

Long-term dialysis access is created via the surgical construction of an AVF or shunt graft. The KDOQI document recommends that the order of preference for the shunt/fistula site should be radiocephalic wrist fistula, followed by brachiocephalic elbow fistula, and transposed brachial–basilic vein fistula. An arteriovenous graft should only be considered if AVF creation is not possible.

Regular assessment of AVFs should be performed to detect hemodynamically significant stenosis, to decrease the incidence of thrombosis of fistula, and to improve long-term patency. Direct flow measurements and duplex ultrasound are preferred methods of surveillance. If there is a decrease in flow rates, intervention with fistulogram is warranted.

## DIALYSIS FISTULAS AND DIALYSIS ARTERIOVENOUS GRAFT

A. **Indications**
   1. **Diagnostic fistulogram** to assess maturation of atriovenous fistula; usually performed 6 weeks after the creation of the fistula.
   2. **Therapeutic fistulogram** assessment of malfunctioning fistula due to anastomotic stenosis, venous outflow stenosis, or fistula thrombosis.
B. **Contraindications**
   1. Infection.
   2. Right-to-left heart shunt.
C. **Preprocedural care**
   1. Refer to Table 16.3 for preprocedural care.
D. **Anesthesia**
   1. Moderate sedation and local anesthesia.
E. **Intraprocedural care**
   1. Refer to Table 16.4 for basic intraprocedural care.
   2. Patient placed on fluoroscopy table usually in supine position.
   3. Heparin 3,000 units IV is given initially and as needed during the procedure.
   4. Nitroglycerin should be available in case of vasospasm.
   5. Ultrasound is used for initially identifying the access site and then fluoroscopy is used.

## FAST FACTS in a NUTSHELL

> Pulses in the major arteries of the arm should be checked and documented before and after a fistulogram.

F. **Postprocedural care**
   1. Refer to Table 16.5 for postprocedural care.
   2. Volume overload can result from the fluids administered during the procedure, especially in those patients with impaired renal function.
      - Evaluate for shortness of breath and auscultate for lung crackles.
      - Patient may need dialysis for fluid overload.
   3. Other complications:
      - Shortness of breath could be caused by a pulmonary embolism.
      - Arterial embolism in the forearm may occur.
        - Assessment for pulses and limb ischemia is therefore important postprocedure.
      - Contrast reaction, infection, hematoma, or bleeding may occur.
   4. Patient may require dialysis after the procedure depending on labs.
G. **Follow-up/patient education**
   1. Outpatient follow-up in 4 to 6 weeks.

## FAST FACTS in a NUTSHELL

> Patient may require dialysis after the procedure depending on labs and fluid status.

# 20

# Aortic Interventions and Transjugular Intrahepatic Portosystemic Shunt

## Ayman Sawas and Ashwani Kumar Sharma

In this chapter, you will discover:

1. Descriptions of aortic aneurysms
2. Treatments for aortic dissection
3. Pressure measurements during a transjugular intrahepatic portosystemic shunt (TIPSS)

## TIPSS

A. **Introduction**
   1. TIPSS is a percutaneous procedure that creates a vascular shunt between the portal venous system and the systemic venous circulation to alleviate portal hypertension.
   2. In most circumstances, access is obtained in the right internal jugular vein.
   3. The catheter is advanced into the hepatic veins. A venogram can be performed.
   4. A shunt is created between a hepatic vein and a portal vein branch.

B. **Indications**
  1. Prevention of variceal bleeding.
  2. Recurrent cirrhotic ascites.
  3. Pleural effusion due to hepatic disease.
C. **Contraindications**
  1. Right heart failure.
  2. Polycystic liver disease.
  3. Diffuse liver metastasis.
  4. Severe or progressive liver failure.
  5. Hepatic encephalopathy.
  6. Coagulopathy.
  7. Main portal vein thrombosis, inferior vena cava thrombosis, or hepatic vein thrombosis.
  8. Allergy to stent components.
  9. Bacteremia.
D. **Preprocedural care**
  1. Refer to Table 16.3 for preprocedural care.
E. **Anesthesia**
  1. Procedure usually performed with moderate sedation and local anesthesia.
  2. General anesthesia can also be used.
F. **Intraprocedural care**
  1. Refer to Table 16.4 for intraprocedural care.
  2. Patient placed on fluoroscopy table, usually in supine position.
  3. Prophylactic antibiotics, usually ceftriaxone or Zosyn, although alternatives include ciprofloxacin or vancomycin.
  4. Venous access for TIPSS is usually the right internal jugular vein.
  5. Ultrasound is used for vein access, then fluoroscopy during the procedure.
  6. Venography is usually performed during the exam.
  7. Pressure transducer is needed, mounted to the procedural table.
     a. Calibrate to zero prior to the procedure.
     b. Pressure measurements before and after TIPSS creation should include: right atrial, central venous, hepatic vein, and hepatic wedge pressures.
        1.) Right atrial pressure should be less than 10 mmHg.
        2.) Portal systemic pressure gradient should be less than 12 mmHg in variceal bleeding.

> Portal venous pressure is the blood pressure in the hepatic portal vein and is normally between 5 and 10 mmHg.

G. **Postprocedural care**
   1. Refer to Table 16.5 for postprocedural care.
   2. Assess for shortness of breath, as patient may develop pulmonary edema and require diuresis.
   3. Assess for mental status, as these patients have a risk of hepatic encephalopathy.
   4. Patients require at least 24-hour observation post-procedure.
   5. Complications of the procedure include entry site hematoma, fever, contrast-induced nephropathy, hemoperitoneum, hemobilia, gallbladder injury, liver infarction, hepatic encephalopathy, stent thrombosis or stenosis, and recurrent variceal bleeding.
H. **Follow-up/patient education**
   1. Outpatient follow-up in 4 to 6 weeks and an ultrasound exam at 3 months to evaluate the patency of the shunt (TIPSS may become stenosed or occluded).

## AORTIC INTERVENTIONS

A. **Introduction**
   1. Aortic interventions are performed to treat significant pathologies of the aorta, including aortic aneurysm and aortic dissection.
   2. **Aortic aneurysm** is an abnormal local dilatation of the aorta that is greater than 50% of normal: The normal limits for the descending thoracic aorta are 3 to 3.5 cm, while the normal limits for the abdominal aorta are 2 to 3 cm. The most common etiology of aortic aneurysms is atherosclerotic disease; other causes include connective tissue disease, inflammatory disease, infection of the aorta, aortic dissection, and trauma. Aortic aneurysms may rupture and lead to death; therefore, repair

is indicated depending on set guidelines that take into account the risk of rupture.

3. **Aortic dissection** occurs when a defect of the aorta's intima layer allows for blood to flow between the layers of the aortic wall. Two major classification systems for dissection are the Stanford system and the DeBakey system. The Stanford system defines dissection involving the ascending thoracic aorta as Type A, while dissections limited to the descending aorta are Type B. The most common etiology of dissection is hypertension; other causes of dissection include atherosclerotic disease, connective tissue disease, and trauma. Dissections can compromise blood flow to the aortic branch or cause aneurysm formation; repair is indicated for complicated dissections.

4. The treatment for aortic aneurysms and dissection can be surgical, endovascular, and medical management.

5. Endovascular repair can be performed by interventional radiology; it is usually performed by gaining access to a common femoral artery and placing a stent or graft to repair the aortic abnormality. For aortic dissection, fenestration of the dissection flap can also be performed for treatment.

6. The procedure is performed through percutaneous access to the femoral artery with a catheter advanced to the aorta. An aortogram can be performed with contrast injection. The common femoral arteries are usually preferred for access, but the common iliac or the abdominal aorta can be accessed also.

B. **Indications**
   1. Symptomatic aneurysms.
   2. Asymptomatic aneurysms larger than 5.5 cm.
   3. Aneurysms that increase in size by more than 1 cm in a year.
   4. Complicated dissections.

C. **Contraindications**
   1. Allergy to stent material.
   2. Increased risk of infection or seeding the stent by infection.
   3. Inappropriate anatomy for repair.

D. **Preprocedural care**
   1. Refer to Table 16.3 for preprocedural care.

E. **Anesthesia**
   1. General, regional, and local anesthesia.
F. **Intraprocedural care**
   1. Refer to Table 16.4 for intraprocedural care.
   2. Patient is placed on fluoroscopy table usually in supine position.
   3. Somatosensory-evoked potentials and electroencephalography are also used to evaluate for neurological complications. Maintaining normal blood pressure is crucial in cases of aortic dissection. Hypotension increases the risk of spinal cord ischemia.

========================================*FAST FACTS in a NUTSHELL*

The vascular surgery consult team should be involved in the care of the patient in case emergency vascular surgery intervention is indicated.

G. **Postprocedural care**
   1. Refer to Table 16.5 for postprocedural care.
   2. Monitoring in an intensive care unit is required for at least 12 hours postprocedure.
   3. The mean arterial pressure should be maintained over 100 mmHg.
   4. Postprocedural monitoring includes evaluation for signs of stroke, ischemia in the extremities by monitoring pulses in all extremities, and signs of spinal ischemia.
   5. Check access site for bleeding or hematoma.
   6. Bed rest is advised for 2 hours postfemoral arterial puncture.
   7. Complications of the procedure include contrast reaction, contrast-induced nephropathy, infection, pain at the access site, hematoma and bleeding at the arterial puncture site, pseudoaneurysm at the arterial puncture site, back pain, bleeding, stroke, spinal cord ischemia, and death.
H. **Follow-up/patient education**
   1. Outpatient follow-up in 4 to 6 weeks.

# 21

# Thoracentesis, Fallopian Tube Recanalization, Vertebroplasty, and Kyphoplasty

## Ayman Sawas and Ashwani Kumar Sharma

In this chapter, you will discover:

1. Treatments for pleural fluid collection
2. Infertility treatment for fallopian tube occlusion
3. Care of the patient undergoing vertebral procedures

## THORACENTESIS

A. **Introduction**
   1. This procedure allows removal of pleural fluid for diagnostic or therapeutic purposes. It can also be performed for pneumothorax drainage.
   2. When bilateral thoracentesis is desired, one side is performed and patient is monitored for complications prior to performing the procedure on the contralateral side.
   3. A pleural drain catheter can be placed for therapeutic drainage after the procedure.

B. **Indications**
   1. **Diagnostic thoracentesis** is used to obtain a sample for laboratory evaluation in order to determine whether a pleural effusion is malignant, parapneumonic effusion due to infection, or a simple effusion.
   2. **Therapeutic thoracentesis** is indicated for draining significant pleural effusions causing dyspnea or hypoxia.
      • Also performed for draining parapneumonic effusion, hemothorax, or pneumothorax.
C. **Contraindications**
   1. Uncorrectable coagulopathy.
D. **Preprocedural Care**
   1. Refer to Table 16.3 for preprocedural care.
E. **Anesthesia**
   1. Procedure is usually performed with minimal sedation and local anesthesia.
   2. Moderate sedation can also be used.
F. **Intraprocedural care**
   1. Refer to Table 16.4 for intraprocedural care.
   2. Patient is placed in the upright sitting position while leaning on the table.
      a. Alternatively, the patient can be placed in the lateral decubitus position.
      b. In certain cases with pneumothorax or loculated effusion, the procedure may be performed with computed tomography (CT) or fluoroscopy guidance and the patient positioning should be confirmed with the operator.
   3. Ultrasound is usually used for identifying the access site.
      a. A limited ultrasound exam is performed for identification of an optimal fluid pocket and the radiologist marks the entry site, usually at the sixth or seventh intercostal rib space at the midaxillary line or back.
   4. Special attention should be paid to respiratory rate and oxygen saturation due to risk of pneumothorax.
   5. Fluid sample may be aspirated and sent for diagnostic evaluation.
   6. A tunneled pleural catheter can be left in place if long-term drainage is desired.
      a. Parapneumonic and exudative effusions usually require a larger bore drain (at least a 12 to 14 French catheter).

b. Transudative effusions can be drained with an 8 to 10 French catheter.

c. Pleural drains need to be connected to a chest tube system to allow for drainage.

7. Entry site into the thorax is covered with occlusive dressing, such as gauze impregnated with white petroleum jelly.

G. **Postprocedural care**

1. Refer to Table 16.5 for postprocedural care.

2. Special attention should be paid to respiratory rate and oxygen saturation.

   a. Check for dyspnea and lung sounds on physical exam, as patient may develop pneumothorax.

3. Upright chest radiograph is performed to evaluate for pneumothorax.

4. Complications of the procedure include pneumothorax, infection, bleeding, and drainage catheter malfunction.

## FAST FACTS in a NUTSHELL

Drainage of fluid should be limited to a maximum of 1 to 1.5 L of fluid in one day to prevent re-expansion pulmonary edema. The amount of fluid drained during the procedure should be communicated to the receiving nurse.

H. **Follow-up/patient education**

1. Outpatient follow-up in 2 to 4 weeks.

2. Patients with a pleural catheter require instructions on outpatient drainage.

   a. A pleural catheter has a bulb that is compressed and connected to the chest tube for drainage when the patient feels fluid accumulating in the pleural cavity.

   b. The bulb then fills with fluid as it drains.

3. Patients with pleural drains are followed clinically by recording output and by radiograph to determine when the pleural drain can be removed.

# FALLOPIAN TUBE RECANALIZATION

A. **Introduction**
   1. Fallopian tube occlusion causes infertility. Fallopian tube recanalization is a procedural treatment for relieving blockages of the fallopian tubes.
   2. Prior to recanalization, a hysterosalpingogram is performed by inserting the catheter through the cervix and injecting contrast dye in the uterine cavity. Upon confirmation of fallopian tubal occlusion, a second catheter is used to cannulate the fallopian tube.
   3. Hysterosalpingogram is then repeated to check for patency of the fallopian tubes.

B. **Indications**
   1. Infertility due to fallopian tube occlusion.
   2. Recanalization after tubal ligation reversal.

C. **Contraindications**
   1. Pelvic infection.
   2. Intrauterine adhesions.
   3. Distal tubal occlusion.
   4. Pregnancy.

D. **Preprocedural care**
   1. Refer to Table 16.3 for preprocedural care.

E. **Anesthesia**
   1. Procedure is usually performed with minimal sedation. Moderate sedation can be used.

F. **Intraprocedural care**
   1. Refer to Table 16.4 for intraprocedural care.
   2. Prophylaxis antibiotics are usually given.
   3. Patient is placed on fluoroscopy table in lithotomy position.
   4. Vaginal speculum is inserted and cervix is prepped in sterile fashion.

G. **Postprocedural care**
   1. Refer to Table 16.5 for postprocedural care.
   2. Assess for abdominal pain, as severe abdominal pain may indicate a complication such as tubal perforation.
   3. Complications of the procedure include pelvic infection, tubal perforation, and ectopic pregnancy.

H. **Follow-up/patient education**
   1. Outpatient follow-up in 4 to 6 weeks.
   2. Vaginal spotting and cramping for the first 2 days is expected.

3. Patient should not engage in sex or put anything in the vagina for 48 hours postprocedure, including tampons.

(YouTube: **www.youtube.com/watch?v=laR3VTQPZ58**)

# VERTEBROPLASTY AND KYPHOPLASTY

A. **Description**
1. Compression fractures of the spinal vertebra can cause significant back pain.
2. Vertebroplasty is a procedure for stabilizing the vertebra by advancing a needle and injecting cement into the vertebral body.
3. Kyphoplasty is a more involved procedure, with a cannula placed into the vertebral pedicle. Then the cannula is used for drilling of the vertebra to create a channel for ballooning and creating a cavity in the vertebral body. This cavity is then filled with cement.
4. Both procedures are performed with fluoroscopy.
5. Patient should have prior imaging such as spinal radiographs, CT of the spine, or MRI of the spine to determine the target vertebra for treatment.

B. **Indications**
1. Vertebral body compression fracture.

C. **Contraindications**
1. Allergy to cement.
2. Systemic infection or bacteremia.
3. Fractures causing spinal canal compromise or spinal cord myelopathy.
4. Coagulopathy.

D. **Preprocedural care**
1. Refer to Table 16.3 for preprocedural care.

E. **Anesthesia**
1. Procedure usually performed with moderate sedation and local anesthesia.

F. **Intraprocedural care**
1. Refer to Table 16.4 for intraprocedural care.
2. Patient placed on fluoroscopy table, usually in prone position.
3. Prophylactic antibiotics are given with Ancef 1 g intravenously.

4. Special attention to room temperature; cement temperature must adhere to manufacturer's recommendations during procedure.

## FAST FACTS in a NUTSHELL

Keep a small amount of mixed cement material aside to observe when it solidifies; this helps staff to determine when the patient can be moved from the fluoroscopy table.

G. **Postprocedural care**
   1. Refer to Table 16.5 for postprocedural care.
H. **Follow-up**
   1. Complications of the procedure include bleeding, infection, pneumothorax when the procedure involves the thoracic vertebra, nerve damage or motor neuropathy, pulmonary emboli from the cement, and fractures of vertebra adjacent to treated vertebra.

# 22

## Embolization Procedures: General, Hepatic, Pulmonary, and Uterine Artery

### Ayman Sawas and Ashwani Kumar Sharma

In this chapter, you will discover:

1. Types of embolization procedures available
2. General and specific patient care essentials
3. Benefits of interventional radiology (IR) embolization interventions

## TRAUMA AND SOLID ORGAN EMBOLIZATION

A. Introduction
   1. Performed to obstruct blood flow for treatment of an array of diseases and medical conditions, such as hemorrhage from traumatic injury, gastrointestinal bleeding, and vascular malformation.
      a. It can also treat tumors, which are discussed in a separate section.
      b. Venous bleeding is usually treated conservatively and does not require embolization.

> Arterial bleeding can be brisk and cause significant blood loss; these patients may require emergent IR and volume resuscitation.

2. These procedures are performed through percutaneous access into the blood vessels, with the catheter advanced to the vessel of interest.
   a. Contrast is injected to select the vessel of interest, embolization material is deployed into the selected blood vessel, followed by a contrast injection to check for success of the embolization.
3. Different types of embolization material are available, including coils, glue, alcohol, gelatin sponge, and microspheres.
4. An imaging study such as a computed tomography (CT) scan prior to the procedure can identify the bleeding source.
5. Access to the large vessel, such as the femoral artery or femoral vein, is gained depending on the abnormality.

B. **Indications**
1. Vascular injury due to trauma. Hemorrhage of gastrointestinal bleeding and arteriovenous malformations. Hemorrhage may need emergent embolization.
2. Hemorrhage from tumor.
3. Tumor treatment in addition to surgery.
4. Splenic artery embolization for splenomegaly and certain types of hematologic disorders.
5. Renal artery embolization for renal tumors such as angiomyolipoma.
6. Uterine artery embolization for uterine fibroids or neoplasm treatment.
7. Uterine vein embolization for pelvic congestion syndrome.

C. **Contraindications**
1. Hemodynamic instability; unstable trauma patients can be managed surgically or should be stabilized prior to the procedure.
2. Renal insufficiency or solitary kidney is a contraindication in renal artery embolization.

D. **Preprocedural care**
1. Refer to Table 16.3 for preprocedural care.

E. **Anesthesia**
   1. Procedure usually performed with moderate sedation and local anesthesia.
F. **Intraprocedural care**
   1. Refer to Table 16.4 for intraprocedural care.
   2. Patient placed on fluoroscopy table, usually in supine position.
   3. Ultrasound is used for identifying the venous site initially and then fluoroscopy is used.
   4. Heparin is usually mixed with normal saline on the sterile tray.
      a. If the patient is allergic to heparin, then alteplase might be used.
G. **Postprocedural care**
   1. Refer to Table 16.5 for postprocedural care.
   2. Arterial puncture site is observed for hematoma or bleeding prior to patient discharge for 2 hours if closure device is used (6 hours if manual compression is used).
      a. Physician must be notified if there is hematoma or swelling at the site.
   3. Bed rest is advised for 2 hours postfemoral arterial puncture.
   4. If the patient develops bleeding, pressure should be applied at the access site and physician must be notified.
   5. Check distal pulses if embolization is performed in the extremities.
   6. Pain control.
H. **Follow-up/patient education**
   1. Patient follows up with outpatient office in 2 to 6 weeks.
   2. Complications of the procedure include contrast reaction, contrast-induced nephropathy, infection, pain at the access site, hematoma and bleeding at the arterial puncture site, pseudoaneurysm at the arterial puncture site, or distal ischemia when embolization is performed in the extremities.

# RADIOEMBOLIZATION OF HEPATIC MALIGNANCIES

A. **Introduction**
   1. This is an endovascular procedure for the treatment of primary hepatic malignancies or metastatic liver lesions.

2. It is performed through percutaneous access into a femoral artery and catheters are advanced to the hepatic arteries. Contrast is injected to select the vessel of interest.
3. It utilizes particles impregnated with radioactive isotope yttrium-90.
   a. These particles are then injected into the hepatic artery and are carried by blood flow to become trapped in the distal arterioles supplying the tumor.
   b. They emit beta particles, thus irradiating the tumor.
4. Theraspheres and SIR-spheres are two types of particles that are used for treatment.
5. Goal of treatment is to shrink the tumor and preserve normal liver parenchyma and function.
6. Preferred access is through the right femoral artery; left femoral artery can also be used.
7. Patient usually has imaging of liver lesion, such as CT or MRI, prior to the procedure.

B. **Indications**
   1. Unresectable hepatocellular carcinoma.
   2. Metastatic neoplasm to the liver.

C. **Contraindications**
   1. Hepatopulmonary lung shunting of more than 20%.
   2. Uncorrectable coagulopathy.
   3. Poor candidate for chemoembolization.
   4. Pregnancy.
   5. Relative contraindications: Poor hepatic function or biliary obstruction.

D. **Preprocedural care**
   1. Refer to Table 16.3 for preprocedural care.

E. **Anesthesia**
   1. Procedure usually performed with moderate sedation and local anesthesia.

F. **Intraprocedural care**
   1. Refer to Table 16.4 for intraprocedural care.
   2. Ultrasound may be used for identifying the venous site initially and then fluoroscopy.
   3. Radioactive precautions should be in place.

G. **Postprocedural care**
   1. Refer to Table 16.5 for postprocedural care.
   2. Bed rest is advised for 2 hours.
   3. Monitor patients for abdominal pain, nausea, and fever: These are managed conservatively.

Careful monitoring of patient should be done postprocedure for idiosyncratic reaction of chills, rigors, and hypotension. This is managed with supportive care using diphenhydramine, meperidine, and fluid resuscitation.

H. **Follow-up/patient education**

1. Outpatient follow-up in 4 to 6 weeks.
2. Discharge instructions with contact information should be provided. Advise patient to seek medical attention if having swelling at puncture site, fevers, or chills.
3. Complications of the procedure include fatigue, abdominal pain, nausea, fever, contrast reaction, contrast-induced nephropathy, infection, pain at the access site, hematoma, and bleeding at the arterial puncture site.

# EMBOLIZATION OF PULMONARY VASCULAR ABNORMALITIES

A. **Introduction**

1. Pulmonary arteriovenous malformations (PAVMs) are formed by a direct connection between a pulmonary artery and a pulmonary vein without an intervening capillary bed. PAVMs are found with Osler-Weber-Rendu syndrome.
2. These malformations can be asymptomatic yet lead to dyspnea, hemoptysis, brain infection, paradoxical embolization (arterial thrombosis), and high-output heart failure.
3. Embolization can be performed by IR to treat these malformations. The procedure utilizes ultrasound to access the femoral vein. Fluoroscopy is then utilized for advancing a catheter through the cardiac chambers to the pulmonary arteries. Pulmonary artery wedge pressure may be performed. A diagnostic pulmonary angiogram is performed to identify the vascular abnormality and to perform the embolization of the abnormality.

B. **Indications**

1. Pulmonary arteriovenous malformations.

2. Pulmonary arteriovenous shunts.
3. Pulmonary artery aneurysms.

C. **Contraindications**
   1. Contrast dye allergy.
D. **Preprocedural care**
   1. Refer to Table 16.3 for preprocedural care.
E. **Anesthesia**
   1. Procedure usually performed with moderate sedation and local anesthesia.
F. **Intraprocedural care**
   1. Refer to Table 16.4 for intraprocedural care.
   2. Patient placed on fluoroscopy table, usually in supine position.
   3. Special attention should be paid to cardiac rhythm during wire or catheter advancement through the cardiac chambers because this can generate heart arrhythmia.
   4. Right femoral vein is usually used for access.
   5. Prophylactic antibiotics, usually cefazolin 1 g intravenously (IV).
   6. Heparin (3,000 to 5,000 units) is used with embolization.
G. **Postprocedural care**
   1. Refer to Table 16.5 for postprocedural care.
   2. Fever and chest pain are the most common side effects. These can occur several days after the procedure and are managed with nonsteroidal anti-inflammatory medications.
   3. Complications of the procedure include entry site hematoma, contrast-induced nephropathy, contrast reaction, paradoxical embolization, and hemorrhage from the malformation.
H. **Follow-up/patient education**
   1. Advise patient to seek medical attention if having swelling at puncture site, persistent fevers or chills, or worsening hemoptysis.
   2. Outpatient follow-up in 4 to 6 weeks.

# UTERINE ARTERY EMBOLIZATION

A. **Introduction**
   1. Performed to obstruct blood flow in the uterine arteries for treatment of uterine fibroids. The procedure can also be performed to treat uterine bleeding.

2. It is performed through percutaneous access into a common femoral artery with the catheter advanced to the uterine arteries. Contrast is injected to select the vessel of interest. Embolization material is then deployed into the selected blood vessel.

3. Patients undergoing uterine artery embolization usually undergo imaging, such as ultrasound or MRI, in the preprocedural evaluation.

B. **Indications**
   1. Fibroids causing dysfunctional menstrual bleeding.
   2. Fibroids causing pelvic pain or pelvic pressure.
   3. Postpartum hemorrhage.

C. **Contraindications**
   1. Pregnancy is contraindication for fibroid embolization.

D. **Preprocedural care**
   1. Refer to Table 16.3 for basic preprocedural care.
   2. Foley catheter should be placed.

E. **Anesthesia**
   1. Procedure usually performed with moderate sedation and local anesthesia. General anesthesia may be a consideration for some patients.

F. **Intraprocedural care**
   1. Refer to Table 16.4 for basic intraprocedural care.
   2. Patient placed on fluoroscopy table, usually in supine position.
   3. Patient usually receives prophylactic antibiotics such as cefazolin.
   4. Ultrasound may be used for initially identifying the access site and then fluoroscopy.
   5. Heparin (1,000–5,000 units) is usually mixed with normal saline on the sterile tray.

G. **Postprocedural care**
   1. Refer to Table 16.5 for basic postprocedural care.
   2. Pain control is essential. A patient-controlled analgesia pump may be used initially then transitioned to nonsteroidal anti-inflammatory medications prior to discharge.
   3. Foley catheter should be removed 6 to 24 hours postprocedure and documentation of patient's ability to void should be performed prior to discharge.
   4. Nausea is a common side effect and antiemetic medication should be ordered.

H. **Follow-up**
   1. Follow up with IR 1 week after procedure.

2. Follow-up imaging with MRI or ultrasound can be performed 3 months postprocedure to evaluate for treatment response.

3. Complications of the procedure include fibroid passage, contrast reaction, contrast-induced nephropathy, infection, pain at the access site, distal ischemia, and hematoma/bleeding/pseudoaneurysm at the arterial puncture site.

# 23

# Embolization Procedures: Chemoembolization, Gastrointestinal Bleeding, and Varicocele

## Mohammed Mohsin Khadir and Labib H. Syed

In this chapter, you will discover:

1. Use of transcatheter arterial chemoembolization (TACE)
2. Treatment of gastrointestinal (GI) bleeding
3. Indication for varicocele intervention

## CHEMOEMBOLIZATION

A. **Introduction**
   1. TACE is a procedure used to treat tumors by selectively delivering chemotherapy to the lesion followed by occlusion of its blood supply.
   2. Unlike normal liver parenchyma, hepatic tumor lesions depend more on hepatic arterial flow than portal venous flow for blood supply, allowing selective treatment of tumor lesions.
   3. TACE is performed by gaining access to the femoral artery by an introducer kit.

a. An arterial sheath is placed into the femoral artery to maintain access, then a catheter is inserted into the sheath and advanced while performing diagnostic angiograms.

b. The catheter is positioned with the tip in the feeding artery of the tumor, usually a branch of the hepatic artery, and then a chemotherapeutic regimen is infused.

c. An embolic agent is used next to increase localization of the chemotherapy and decrease tumor blood flow to induce ischemic necrosis of the lesion.

## FAST FACTS in a NUTSHELL

Commonly used chemotherapeutic drugs with chemoembolization are cisplatin, doxorubicin, and mitomycin C.

B. **Indications**
1. Used as palliation of unresectable hepatocellular carcinomas.
2. Treatment of lesions can maintain or downstage patients to within liver transplantation criteria.
3. Treatment of metastatic lesions that are primarily confined to the liver.

C. **Contraindications**
1. Poorly compensated advanced liver disease.
2. Poor performance status.
3. Large tumor burden.
4. Untreatable coagulopathy.
5. Severe contrast reaction.

D. **Preprocedural care**
1. Refer to Table 16.3 for preprocedural care.
2. Hypotensive patients should be fluid-resuscitated prior to procedure.
3. Prophylactic antibiotics are given.

E. **Anesthesia**
1. Chemoembolization is performed under conscious sedation.

F. **Intraprocedural care**
1. Refer to Table 16.4 for intraprocedural care.
2. Place patient in supine position.

3. Access site is usually the right femoral artery.
4. Prepare chemotherapeutic drugs for the physician.
5. Prepare embolic agent, typically embolization spheres.

G. **Postprocedure care**
   1. Refer to Table 16.5 for postprocedural care.
   2. Patients are placed on a patient-controlled analgesia (PCA) pump to control postoperative pain.
   3. Patient may be given intravenous (IV) fluids and antiemetics.

H. Complications
   1. Liver failure may occur in patients with poor preprocedure liver function.
      a. Monitor for signs of encephalopathy, coagulopathy, and renal failure.
      b. These may be managed with fluids, pressure support, and lactulose.
   2. Nontarget embolization of the gut, which can lead to bowel ischemia.

I. **Follow-up/patient education**
   1. Patients follow up with interventional radiologist in 4 to 6 weeks GI

# GI BLEEDING

A. **Introduction**
   1. Acute GI bleeding can be suspected to originate from the **upper GI tract** when a patient presents with hematemesis and/or black tarry stools.
      a. If the bleeding is brisk, hypotension and tachycardia will be present and resuscitative efforts will be essential.
      b. Diagnosis and treatment of the bleeding vessels are attempted first by a gastroenterologist using an endoscope. If unsuccessful, an interventional radiologist may be requested to localize and embolize the target vessel.
   2. For bleeding suspected to originate from the **lower GI tract**, endoscopy is passed over for embolization techniques.
      a. Embolization of the bleeding vessels is performed by gaining access to the femoral artery and an arterial sheath is placed to maintain access. A catheter is inserted into the sheath and advanced into the aorta while performing diagnostic angiograms.

    b. The celiac trunk and the superior mesenteric artery branches are investigated in detail because the target artery is usually a branch from one of these vessels. If a bleeding artery is found, it is then infused with an embolic agent until flow in the artery ceases.

B. **Indications**
1. Bleeding from the upper GI tract that cannot be remedied with an endoscope.
2. Lower GI tract bleeding.

C. **Contraindications**
1. No absolute contraindications when bleeding is life-threatening.
2. Relative contraindications include renal insufficiency, contrast allergy, and untreatable coagulopathy.

D. **Preprocedural care**
1. Refer to Table 16.3 for preprocedural care.
2. Hypotensive patients should be fluid-resuscitated prior to procedure, if acuity permits.

E. **Anesthesia**
1. Embolization is performed under conscious sedation or general anesthesia.

F. **Intraprocedural care**
1. Refer to Table 16.4 for basic intraprocedural care.
2. Patient is placed in supine position.

G. **Postprocedural care**
1. Refer to Table 16.5 for basic postprocedural care.
2. Regular checks of lower-extremity pulses to assess for distal embolization.
3. Vital sign trend demonstrating hypotension and/or tachycardia is suspect for ongoing hemorrhage.
4. Patients may be placed on a PCA pump to control post-procedural pain.

H. **Complications**
1. Nontarget embolization of the gut or other organs rarely leads to ischemia due to rich collateral supply in the abdomen.

I. **Follow-up/patient education**
1. Patient follows up with primary care physician after procedure.
2. Discharge instructions with contact information should be provided.

Nasogastric and stool output should be monitored for gross blood, which might present even though bleeding has stopped because of residual blood in the gastrointestinal tract.

## VARICOCELE

A. **Introduction**
   1. Varicocele is a tortuous dilatation of the pampiniform venous plexus in the scrotum due to incompetent valves in the internal spermatic vein.
   2. The condition presents with dull, aching scrotal pain that frequently only affects the left side. The entity is associated with dysfunctional sperm and is more frequently detected in infertile men.
   3. Treated by embolizing the internal spermatic vein.
   4. Varicocele embolization is performed by gaining access to the right femoral vein or right internal jugular vein. A wire is then placed and a catheter is advanced to the internal spermatic vein. The target vessel is then occluded using embolization coils or foam.

B. **Indications**
   1. Scrotal pain.
   2. Infertility.
   3. Recurrent varicocele.
   4. Testicular atrophy in pediatric patients.

C. **Contraindications**
   1. Severe coagulopathy.
   2. Severe contrast reaction.

D. **Preprocedural care**
   1. Refer to Table 16.3 for preprocedural care.

E. **Anesthesia**
   1. Varicocele embolization is performed under conscious sedation.

F. **Intraprocedural care**
   1. Refer to Table 16.4 for intraprocedural care.
   2. Place patient in supine position.

    3. Ultrasound may be used for initially identifying the vein and then fluoroscopy is used.

G. **Postprocedural care**

    1. Refer to Table 16.5 for postprocedural care.

H. **Complications**

    1. A small percentage of patients will develop:

       a. Back pain that can be treated with acetaminophen.

       b. Scrotal edema that can be managed with nonsteroidal anti-inflammatory drugs and a heating pad.

    2. Migration of embolization coils into the central venous system and venous perforation, which is usually self-limiting.

I. **Follow-up/patient education**

    1. Patient follows up with primary care physician after procedure.

    2. Discharge instructions with contact information should be provided.

# Biliary Procedures

## Labib H. Syed and Mohammed Mohsin Khadir

In this chapter, you will discover:

1. The difference in diagnostic versus therapeutic biliary procedures
2. Common complications of biliary procedures
3. Biliary catheter care

## PERCUTANEOUS TRANSHEPATIC CHOLANGIOGRAPHY (PTC)

A. **Introduction**
   1. PTC is a diagnostic procedure that is performed under fluoroscopy and allows for the visualization and evaluation of the intrahepatic and extrahepatic bile ducts.
   2. PTC is performed by first puncturing the skin overlying the liver with a 21- or 22-gauge needle. Ultrasound is used to assess the anatomical structures and to select a puncture site. The needle is advanced under fluoroscopic guidance using a contrast agent to visualize and access the biliary tract.

B. **Indications**
1. Performed to evaluate the biliary system for dilatation, stenosis, or an obstruction.
C. **Contraindications**
1. Untreatable coagulopathy.
2. Recent antiplatelet agent use.
3. Relative contraindications include large-volume ascites.
D. **Preprocedural care**
1. Refer to Table 16.3 for preprocedural care.
2. Prophylactic antibiotics are given.
E. **Anesthesia**
1. Performed with conscious sedation.
F. **Intraprocedural care**
1. Refer to Table 16.4 for intraprocedural care.
2. Place patient in supine position and prep the right upper quadrant of the abdomen.
G. **Postprocedure care**
1. Refer to Table 16.5 for postprocedural care.
H. **Complications**
1. Subcapsular hematoma or peritoneal bleeding.
   a. Monitor for discomfort, hypotension, and tachycardia.
2. Peritonitis may develop from a bile leak.
   a. Monitor for abdominal pain, tenderness, and guarding.
I. **Follow-up/patient education**
1. Patient follows up with primary care physician after procedure.

## PERCUTANEOUS BILIARY DRAINAGE

A. **Introduction**
1. A therapeutic procedure performed to drain bile from the biliary system.
2. The first part of the procedure is identical to a percutaneous transhepatic cholangiogram. After access is gained and a cholangiogram is performed, a wire is passed into the needle and guided into the bile ducts, and a locking pigtail catheter is placed with the tip curled in the duodenum. The catheter is sutured to the skin, a drainage bag is connected, and dressings are applied.
B. **Indications**
1. This procedure allows for the removal of bile in cases of obstruction, biliary infection, and bile leaks.

C. **Contraindications**
   1. No absolute contraindications.
   2. Relative contraindications include untreatable coagulopathy, recent antiplatelet agent use, and large-volume ascites.
D. **Preprocedural care**
   1. Refer to Table 16.3 for preprocedural care.
   2. Prophylactic antibiotics are given.
   3. Ultrasound is used to evaluate liver and determine access site.
E. **Anesthesia**
   1. Percutaneous biliary drainage is performed with conscious sedation.
F. **Intraprocedural care**
   1. Refer to Table 16.4 for basic intraprocedural care.
   2. Place patient in supine position and prep the right upper quadrant of the abdomen.
G. **Postprocedural care**
   1. Refer to Table 16.5 for basic postprocedural care.
   2. Dressing changes should be performed daily.
   3. Drainage from the catheter should be recorded every 8 hours.
H. **Complications**
   1. Monitor for leakage around the catheter, signs of infection at the skin site, or if a significant change in output occurs (notify physician).
   2. Sepsis, although rare, can occur from the procedure.
      a. Monitor for change in vital signs (increasing temperature and heart rate, decreasing blood pressure) and notify physician.
   3. As with a PTC, patients can develop a subcapsular hematoma, peritoneal bleeding, or peritonitis from a bile leak.
I. **Follow-up/patient education**
   1. Catheter is removed by a radiologist when the primary care physician considers it appropriate.
   2. Patient should contact primary care physician if puncture site demonstrates signs of infection.

*FAST FACTS in a NUTSHELL*

The catheter should be flushed with 10 cc of normal saline if drainage stops, or flushed daily if the catheter is capped.

# PERCUTANEOUS CHOLECYSTOSTOMY

A. **Introduction**
   1. Percutaneous cholecystostomy is a therapeutic procedure that is performed to drain the gallbladder by placing a catheter into its lumen.
   2. Ultrasound is used to assess the anatomy and select a puncture site in the right upper abdomen. The gallbladder is then accessed using a trocar catheter or a sheathed needle. A floppy wire is then passed through the needle into the gallbladder. A tract is created and a locking pigtail catheter is placed with the tip curled in the gallbladder. Bile fluid samples are removed for gram stain and culture.

B. **Indications**
   1. Typically performed in acute patients who are poor surgical candidates.

C. **Contraindications**
   1. No absolute contraindications.
   2. Relative contraindications include untreatable coagulopathy, recent antiplatelet agent use, and large-volume ascites.

D. **Preprocedural care**
   1. Refer to Table 16.3 for preprocedural care.
   2. Prophylactic antibiotics are given.

E. **Anesthesia**
   1. Performed with conscious sedation.

F. **Intraprocedural care**
   1. Refer to Table 16.4 for intraprocedural care.
   2. Place patient in supine position and prep the right upper quadrant of the abdomen.

G. **Postprocedural care**
   1. Refer to Table 16.5 for postprocedural care.
   2. Dressing changes should be performed daily.
   3. Drainage from the catheter should be recorded every 8 hours.

H. **Complications**
   1. Monitor for leakage around the catheter, signs of infection at the skin site, or a significant change in output (notify physician).
   2. Major complications include bile leak leading to peritonitis, bleeding, and sepsis.

I. Follow-up/patient education
   1. Catheter is removed by a radiologist when the primary care physician considers it appropriate.
   2. Patient should contact primary care physician if puncture site demonstrates signs of infection.

*FAST FACTS in a NUTSHELL*

Flush the catheter with 10 cc of normal saline every 6 to 8 hours or if drainage stops.

# 25

# Abscess Drainage, Percutaneous Biopsies, and Nephrostomy Tube

## Mohammed Mohsin Khadir and Labib H. Syed

In this chapter, you will discover:

1. How an abscess is drained
2. The process to biopsy tissue
3. Indication for a nephrostomy tube placement

## ABSCESS DRAINAGE

A. **Introduction**
   1. Percutaneous technique used for abscess drainage offers many advantages to traditional open surgical drainage and has become the first-line therapy in treating infected fluid collections.
   2. If the abscess is located superficially, the procedure is straightforward.
      a. Deeper locations can present as a challenge due to increased risk for injury to the surrounding structures.
   3. The procedure can be performed under ultrasound, computed tomography (CT), or fluoroscopic guidance.
      a. The most appropriate modality and optimal tract to the collection is determined by the location and nature of the collection.

4. Small collections are aspirated and the collected samples are sent to the lab for analysis. Frequently ordered tests include gram stain and culture.

5. Larger collections are accessed with a needle followed by creation of a tract and placement of a locking pigtail catheter, which is then sutured to the skin and attached to a drainage bag with a three-way stopcock.

B. **Indications**
   1. Percutaneous abscess drainage can be diagnostic and/or therapeutic.

C. **Contraindications**
   1. No absolute contraindications.

D. **Preprocedural care**
   1. Refer to Table 16.3 for preprocedural care.
   2. Give prophylactic antibiotics to prevent infection if deemed necessary by physician.

E. **Anesthesia**
   1. Local anesthesia for small collections and conscious sedation for larger collections.

F. **Intraprocedural care**
   1. Refer to Table 16.4 for intraprocedural care.
   2. Patient is positioned on the procedural table in a variety of manners depending on the characteristics of the collection. The position is determined by the physician.

G. **Postprocedural care**
   1. Refer to Table 16.5 for postprocedural care.
   2. Drainage from the catheter should be recorded every 8 hours.
   3. Drainage should decrease daily and the catheter removed when less than 20 cc per day of fluid is returned.
   4. Poor output or occlusion of the catheter can be remedied with tissue plasminogen activator infusion.

H. **Complications**
   1. Hemorrhage, sepsis, and peritonitis.
   2. If there is an increase in fluid drainage, especially greater than 50 cc of fluid per day, the patient might have developed a fistula. Notify the physician.

I. **Follow-up/patient education**
   1. Catheter is removed by a radiologist when the primary care physician considers it appropriate.
   2. Patient should contact primary care physician if puncture site demonstrates signs of infection.

> When a drainage catheter is placed, the catheter should be flushed toward the collection and toward the drainage bag with 10 cc of normal saline every 8 hours to prevent occlusion.

## PERCUTANEOUS BIOPSY

A. **Introduction**
   1. One of the most common procedures performed by interventional radiologists.
   2. A tissue sample from the target lesion can differentiate a benign from malignant process and identify the type of benign or malignant process occurring.
   3. Common structures biopsied percutaneously include the thyroid, superficial skin and muscle structures, lungs, abdominal organs, pelvic organs, lymph nodes, and bone.
   4. The type and location of the target lesion will determine the imaging modality utilized: ultrasound, fluoroscopy, CT, or MRI.
   5. Percutaneous biopsies can be performed with a variety of needles depending on the location and the type of lesion suspected. After access is gained to the target tissue, several passes are made to ensure an adequate sample is taken. The sample is placed in a formalin container and sent to the pathology department.
B. **Indication**
   1. Percutaneous biopsies are performed on sample tissue.
C. **Contraindication**
   1. No absolute contraindications.
   2. Relative contraindications include uncorrectable coagulopathy.
D. **Preprocedural care**
   1. Refer to Table 16.3 for preprocedural care.
E. **Anesthesia**
   1. Percutaneous biopsies are performed with local anesthesia; conscious sedation can be used if necessary.
F. **Intraprocedural care**
   1. Refer to Table 16.4 for intraprocedural care.

G. **Postprocedural care**
   1. Refer to Table 16.5 for basic postprocedural care.
H. **Complications**
   2. The most common, although rare, complications are bleeding and infection.
I. **Follow-up/patient education**
   1. Patient follows up with primary care physician after procedure.
   2. Patient should contact primary care physician if puncture site demonstrates signs of infection.

# PERCUTANEOUS NEPHROSTOMY TUBE PLACEMENT

A. **Introduction**
   1. Drain the upper urinary tract in cases of acute or chronic obstructive uropathy.
   2. Patients can develop a urinary tract obstruction for various reasons, from stones to tumors, and timely placement of a nephrostomy tube can prove essential in maintaining renal function and preventing urosepsis.
   3. Other indications for a percutaneous nephrostomy tube include access to the urinary tract for interventions and to divert urine in cases of a urine leak or urinoma.
   4. During tube placement, ultrasound is used to assess the anatomy and select the optimal approach to the kidney. The renal collecting system is accessed with a puncture needle, a wire is fed through the needle, and a tract is created for placement of a locking pigtail catheter. The catheter tip is curled in the renal pelvis and the free end is sutured to the skin.
B. **Indications**
   1. Obstructive uropathy.
   2. Urinary diversion.
   3. Percutaneous access for interventions.
   4. Pyonephrosis.
C. **Contraindications**
   1. Untreatable coagulopathy.
D. **Preprocedural care**
   1. Refer to Table 16.3 for preprocedural care.

E. **Anesthesia**
  1. Percutaneous nephrostomy tube placement is performed with conscious sedation.
F. **Intraprocedural care**
  1. Refer to Table 16.4 for intraprocedural care.
  2. Patient is positioned in prone position.
  3. Prophylactic antibiotics are administered.
G. **Postprocedural care**
  1. Refer to Table 16.5 for postprocedural care.
  2. Fluid intake and urine output should be recorded. Blood-tinged urine can occur for the first 48 hours postprocedure, but frank hematuria should not be present.
  3. The catheter should be flushed every 4 hours with 5 cc of normal saline if clots are present.
H. **Complications**
  1. Major complications from the procedure include massive hemorrhage, injury to surrounding organs, or sepsis.
  2. Patients with hemorrhage can present with hypotension and may require surgery or embolization to control the bleeding.
  3. Minor complications include a urine leak and pain at the procedure site.
I. **Follow-up/patient education**
  1. Catheter is removed by a radiologist when the primary care physician considers it appropriate.
  2. Patient should contact primary care physician if puncture site demonstrates signs of infection.

# 26

# Paracentesis and Gastrostomy Tube

## Mohammed Mohsin Khadir and Labib H. Syed

In this chapter, you will discover:

1. Purpose of paracentesis
2. Care of the patient during procedure
3. Process for G-tube placement

## PARACENTESIS

A. **Introduction**
   1. Paracentesis involves the removal of fluid accumulated in the peritoneal cavity for diagnostic or therapeutic purposes.
   2. Peritoneal fluid is analyzed to diagnose infection or metastasis to the peritoneal cavity.
      a. Tests may include cell count, cell differential, albumin, lactate dehydrogenase, and cultures.
   3. A therapeutic paracentesis relieves tense ascites, commonly occurring in cirrhotic patients.
      a. A larger-gauge needle is used to remove as much fluid as tolerated by the patient.
      b. Several different needles can be used; typically an 18-gauge is preferred.

       c. Newer devices include a one-step needle, which has a removable needle inside a catheter, and a valved one-step needle.

    4. The procedure can be performed at bedside or in the radiology department (for more complicated patients).

B. **Indications**

    1. Evaluation of new-onset ascites.

    2. Diagnostic testing in patients with signs of an infection of the peritoneal cavity such as fever, abdominal pain, abdominal tenderness, leukocytosis.

    3. Testing of peritoneal fluid in patients with preexisting ascites.

C. **Contraindications**

    1. If benefits outweigh the risks, paracentesis is always performed.

    2. Relative contraindications include disseminated intravascular coagulation and massive ileus with bowel distention.

    3. Elevated international normalized ratio or coagulopathy is not a contraindication for paracentesis.

D. **Preprocedural care**

    1. Refer to Table 16.3 for basic preprocedural care.

E. **Anesthesia**

    1. Typically performed with local anesthesia, but can use conscious sedation.

F. **Intraprocedural care**

    1. Refer to Table 16.4 for intraprocedural care.

    2. Place patient in supine position.

    3. Ultrasound is performed for identification of the optimal fluid pocket.

    4. Radiologist marks the entry site, usually in the left lower abdominal quadrant.

    5. Peritoneal fluid collected for analysis should be labeled per organization policy.

G. **Special considerations**

    1. Start colloid replacement with a 5% or 25% solution after 3 to 5 liters of fluid are removed.

    2. Patients not receiving albumin are more likely to show signs of hemodynamic deterioration and worsening renal function.

If more than 3 to 5 liters of fluid are removed, 6 to 8 g of albumin for every liter of fluid removed is given to prevent hypotension.

H. **Postprocedural care**
1. Refer to Table 16.5 for postprocedural care.
I. **Complications**
1. Leakage of peritoneal fluid, infection, bleeding, and injury to bowel.
2. For a peritoneal fluid leak, an occlusive dressing or topical adhesive can be applied.
   a. If the leak continues, an ostomy bag can be placed to quantify the fluid and further treatment options can be discussed with a physician.
   b. Intraperitoneal infections from the procedure are rare; a persistent leak can lead to cellulitis at the puncture site.
3. Bleeding from an injured artery or vein can be severe.
   a. Abdomen pain, tenderness, and hypotension should raise concern.
J. **Follow-up/patient education**
1. Patient follows up with primary care physician after procedure.
2. Patient should contact primary care physician if puncture site demonstrates signs of infection or if the fluid reaccumulates.

## GASTROSTOMY TUBE

A. **Introduction**
1. Gastrostomy and gastrojejunostomy tubes are placed to provide enteric access for long-term nutritional goals.
2. A gastrostomy tube has one tip positioned in the gastric lumen, while a gastrojejunostomy tube has an additional tip inserted distally in the jejunum.

a. A gastrojejunostomy tube is preferred over a gastrostomy tube if the patient has an aspiration risk, gastric motility problems, or a gastric outlet obstruction.

b. Radiologists utilize a percutaneous method for tube placement, but an endoscopic or surgical technique can also be used for tube placement.

c. Intraprocedurally, a nasogastric tube is used to insufflate the stomach to bring the gastric and abdominal walls flush with each other.

B. **Indications**
   1. Nutritional support.
   2. Diversion of feeding from esophagus in the setting of esophageal surgery or trauma.
   3. Decompression of gastroenteric contents with a need for jejunal feedings.

C. **Contraindications**
   1. No proper percutaneous route to stomach.
   2. Uncorrectable coagulopathy.
   3. Relative contraindications include altered gastric anatomy from prior surgeries and massive ascites.

D. **Preprocedural care**
   1. Refer to Table 16.3 for preprocedural care.
   2. Hypotensive patients should have fluid resuscitated prior to procedure.
   3. Barium may be administered the night before placement to assist with imaging during the procedure.

E. **Anesthesia**
   1. Tube placement is performed under conscious sedation.

F. **Intraprocedural care**
   1. Refer to Table 16.4 for intraprocedural care.
   2. Place patient in supine position.
   3. Glucagon 1 mg intravenously is administered to diminish gastric peristalsis.

G. **Postprocedural care**
   1. Refer to Table 16.5 for postprocedural care.
   2. The tube will be clamped for the first 24 hours postprocedure.

h. **Complications**
   1. Monitor patient for a leaking catheter, peritonitis, or hemorrhage.
   2. A dysfunctional tube should be evaluated by a physician.
   3. Peritonitis presents as abdominal pain, tenderness, and guarding.

4. Hemorrhage presents with abdominal pain and hypotension.

4. Hemorrhage presents with abdominal pain and hypotension.
5. Monitor for reflux, aspiration, or bloating.

I. **Follow-up/patient education**
1. Gastrostomy tube is evaluated by a radiologist 24 hours after placement.
2. Regular tube checks are scheduled at 4- to 6-month intervals.
3. Patient should be informed to contact primary care physician if tube is not functioning properly.

━━━━━━━━━━━━━━━━━━━━ *FAST FACTS in a NUTSHELL*

Initial tube feedings are started at 10 cc/hour and increased to a goal as set by the physician.

# 27

## Ablation and Peripheral Arterial Disease

### Mohammed Mohsin Khadir and Labib H. Syed

In this chapter, you will discover:

1. The difference between thermal ablation and cryoablation
2. Symptoms of peripheral artery disease
3. Treatment of peripheral artery disease

## CRYOABLATION OR RADIOFREQUENCY ABLATION

A. **Introduction**
  1. Minimally invasive techniques of radiofrequency ablation and cryoablation have gained acceptance in the treatment of small tumor lesions.
  2. **Thermal energy** is utilized with radiofrequency ablation and extremely **cold temperatures** with cryoablation to destroy the target lesion.
  3. These minimally invasive techniques offer the benefit of preservation of organ function, shorter recovery time, and reduced mortality and morbidity.
  4. **Radiofrequency ablation:** A needle electrode is advanced under imaging guidance until it reaches the proper position in the target tissue. A heat generator connected to

the needle is used to increase temperatures at the uninsulated tip with a goal of 60°C to 100°C for a proper amount of time. Several passes are taken if the lesion is larger than the probe's ablation diameter.

5. **Cryoablation:** Hollow needles are placed simultaneously into the target tissue, with larger tumors requiring more needles. Liquid argon or carbon dioxide is then used to rapidly cool the uninsulated tip to -100°C to -190°C for a set amount of time. Several cycles of freezing, thawing, and refreezing occur.

6. Typical candidates for these procedures are patients with several small lesions or patients with comorbidities precluding traditional surgical resection.

7. Interventional radiologists usually treat tumors located in the liver or kidney with these procedures, but breast, prostate, and lung lesions can also be treated.

B. **Indications**
   1. Palliative care for hepatocellular carcinoma.
   2. Treatment of liver metastasis.

C. **Contraindications**
   1. Tumor lesion located close to a main biliary duct.
   2. Intrahepatic biliary duct dilation.
   3. Untreatable coagulopathy.

D. **Preprocedural care**
   1. Refer to Table 16.3 for preprocedural care.

E. **Anesthesia**
   1. Radiofrequency ablation and cryoablation are performed under general anesthesia.

F. **Intraprocedural care**
   1. Refer to Table 16.4 for intraprocedural care.
   2. Check with physician for patient positioning. Ablation typically performed with patient in prone position.
   3. Ultrasound or computed tomography (CT) guidance is used to determine the best approach to the tumor.

G. **Postprocedural care**
   1. Refer to Table 16.5 for postprocedural care.
   2. Bed rest is advised for 2 hours and the patient is monitored as an inpatient for 24 hours.
   3. Monitor urine output.
      a. If there is patient discomfort, inability to urinate, or no urine output for 8 hours postsurgery, consider a bedside bladder scan.
      b. Physician may order the placement of a urinary catheter.

H. **Complications**
1. Minor side effects from the procedure include pain at the ablation site and fever.
2. Major complications may include:
   a. Intraperitoneal hemorrhage (abdominal pain, tenderness, hypotension).
   b. Intestinal perforation (rigid abdomen with tenderness).
   c. Pneumothorax (shortness of breath).
I. **Follow-up/patient education**
1. Follow-up with the interventional radiologist in 4 to 6 weeks.
2. Patient should contact the primary care physician if puncture site demonstrates signs of infection, or if there is swelling at puncture site, fevers, or chills.

═══════════════════════════════════*FAST FACTS in a NUTSHELL*

A rare complication of cryoablation is cryoshock, which can result in disseminated intravascular coagulopathy and multisystem organ failure.

# PERIPHERAL ARTERIAL DISEASE (PAD)

A. **Introduction**
1. PAD is defined as compromised blood flow to the extremities due to atherosclerotic calcifications of the feeding vessels.
2. Symptoms develop when there is an imbalance between blood supply and demand.
3. Mild disease presents with reproducible discomfort and pain in a group of muscles upon exertion that resolves with rest.
4. Severe disease leads to pain even at rest and ischemic skin lesions, such as ulcerations.
5. Treatment begins with lifestyle modifications and medical therapy before resorting to interventional therapies.
6. Common minimally invasive revascularization techniques include angioplasty and stenting to improve flow to the distal extremity. Access is gained to the femoral artery and a sheath is placed into the femoral artery to maintain access. A catheter is inserted into the sheath and a runoff angiogram of the lower extremity

is performed to determine areas of stenosis/occlusion. The area is then treated with balloon angioplasty or stent placement.

B. **Indications**
   1. Peripheral arterial disease refractory to lifestyle and medical management.
   2. Critical limb ischemia.

C. **Contraindications**
   1. Uncorrectable coagulopathy.
   2. Allergy to metal in stent.
   3. Allergy to contrast dye.

D. **Preprocedural care**
   1. Refer to Table 16.3 for preprocedural care.

E. **Anesthesia**
   1. The procedure is performed with conscious sedation.

F. **Intraprocedural care**
   1. Refer to Table 16.4 for intraprocedural care.
   2. Place patient in supine position.
   3. Access site is usually the right femoral artery.

G. **Postprocedural care**
   1. Refer to Table 16.5 for postprocedural care.
   2. Regular checks of lower extremity pulses and ankle–brachial index are performed to assess for distal embolization.
   3. May be placed on a patient-controlled analgesia pump to control postoperative pain.

H. **Complications**
   1. May include emboli, pseudoaneurysm, or hematoma formation.
   2. Embolization of the atherosclerotic plaque presents with pain and diminished pulses distal to the site of intervention.
   3. Some patients may have a cool and painful foot with strong pulses.

I. **Follow-up/patient education**
   1. Patient follow-up with primary care physician after procedure.

## FAST FACTS in a NUTSHELL

A tender pulsatile mass at the puncture site in the groin should prompt evaluation for a pseudoaneurysm.

# Filters and Foreign Bodies

## Ayman Sawas and Ashwani Kumar Sharma

In this chapter, you will discover:

1. The process to retrieve foreign bodies utilizing interventional radiology (IR) services
2. Indications for inferior vena cava (IVC) filter placement
3. Types of IVC filters available

## VENA CAVAL FILTERS

A. Introduction
1. These devices are usually placed in the IVC to prevent pulmonary embolism by trapping a thrombus that can break from lower-extremity thrombi or placed in the superior vena cava (SVC) for patients with upper-extremity deep vein thrombosis (DVT).
2. Pulmonary embolism or deep venous thrombi are usually treated pharmacologically with anticoagulation therapy. Vena cava filters are employed in cases where there is a contraindication for pharmacological treatment such as bleeding, in cases of failed anticoagulation therapy, or in cases of large clot burden.

3. These filters can also be used prophylactically in patients with high risk for developing DVT, such as trauma or surgical patients that will be immobilized for an extensive length of time.
4. There are three main categories of filters:
   a. Permanent filters
      1.) Placed permanently and are not intended to be removed or repositioned.
   b. Optional filters
      1.) Filters designed so that they can be retrieved if desired.
   c. Temporary filters
      1.) Filters that have to be removed.
         – Optional and temporary filters are more commonly used, and the Society of Interventional Radiology recommends removal of these filters.
         – Different manufacturer types of these filters exist and they vary by design and delivery system, including vein for access.

B. **Indications**
   1. Documented DVT or patients at high risk for developing DVT with inability to properly treat with pharmacological therapy.
C. **Contraindications**
   1. Total thrombosis of the vena cava.
   2. Lack of access or imaging for delivery of the filter.
   3. Allergy to filter components.
   4. Bacteremia.
D. **Preprocedural care**
   1. Refer to Table 16.3 for preprocedural care.
E. **Anesthesia**
   1. Procedure is usually performed with moderate sedation and local anesthesia.
F. **Intraprocedural care**
   1. Refer to Table 16.4 for intraprocedural care.
   2. Patient placed on fluoroscopy table, usually in supine position.
   3. Ultrasound may be used for identifying the venous site initially and then fluoroscopy.
   4. Venous access for placement of filter can be the common femoral veins or the jugular veins. A direct approach into the SVC can also be performed.

5. Venography is performed during the exam to assess for proper placement of filter.

G. **Postprocedural care**
   1. Refer to Table 16.5 for postprocedural care.
   2. Assess lower extremities for increased swelling, which can indicate clotting of IVC filter.
   3. Complications of the procedure include contrast reaction; contrast-induced nephropathy; entry site hematoma; infection; lower-extremity edema; recurrent pulmonary embolism; cava thrombosis; and filter migration, fracture, or failure.

---

### FAST FACTS in a NUTSHELL

Be sure patient receives product information, including name of product, model, and lot number for the filter placed. The patient may need this information in the future when having an MRI, if there is a product recall from the company, or if complications occur.

H. **Follow-up/patient education**
   1. Outpatient follow-up in 4 to 6 weeks.
   2. Retrievable filters: Venous Doppler ultrasound is scheduled to assess for remaining venous thrombus prior to filter removal. Follow-up appointment for removal of the filter is determined by the patient's need for the filter and the manufacturer's recommendation for retrieval.
   3. Permanent filters: Abdominal radiographs every 3 to 4 years to evaluate filter position and integrity.

## VENA CAVAL FILTER RETRIEVAL

A. **Introduction**
   1. The new types of vena cava filters are designed to be removed.
      a. Removal is recommended and reduces the risk of filter-related complications.

2. Access into a large vein, such as the internal jugular vein or femoral vein, is gained depending on the filter design.
3. Cavogram is performed by advancing a catheter and injecting contrast to visualize the vena cava.
4. Sheath and snare are utilized to remove the filter. DVT is usually performed.

B. **Indications**
1. Filter is no longer needed due to adequate venous thrombus therapy.
2. Patient is no longer at a risk for venous thromboembolism.
3. Filter fails to offer protection against venous thromboembolism due to structural failure or filter migration.
4. Filter causing pain.

C. **Contraindications**
1. Persistent DVT or retained thrombus within the filter.
2. Patient remains at high risk for venous thrombus embolism.
3. Lack of venous access for filter retrieval.
4. Terminal illness with less than 6-month life expectancy.

D. **Preprocedural care**
1. Refer to Table 16.3 for preprocedural care.

E. **Anesthesia**
1. Procedure usually performed with moderate sedation and local anesthesia.

F. **Intraprocedural care**
1. Refer to Table 16.4 for intraprocedural care.
2. Patient placed on fluoroscopy table, usually in supine position.
3. Ultrasound maybe used for initially identifying the venous site and then fluoroscopy.

G. **Postprocedural care**
1. Refer to Table 16.5 for postprocedural care.

H. **Complications**
1. Complications include contrast reaction, contrast-induced nephropathy, infection, and pain at the access site.

I. **Follow-up/patient education**
1. Patient follows up with primary care physician after procedure.
2. Therapy and prophylaxis for venous thrombosis can be resumed and continued until no longer clinically needed.

A. **Introduction**
   1. Foreign bodies can be dislodged and it may be necessary to remove them.
      a. Such scenarios include broken intravascular catheters, wires, nonvascular catheters, stents, or other foreign bodies.
   2. Procedure for removal of these bodies depends on the location and the type of body.
   3. Snares, forceps, and other instruments can be utilized to remove these bodies.
   4. Imaging demonstrating these foreign bodies is usually performed prior to the procedure.
B. **Indications**
   1. Foreign body posing a significant risk to the patient.
C. **Contraindications**
   1. Case-dependent.
D. **Preprocedural care**
   1. Refer to Table 16.3 for preprocedural care.
E. **Anesthesia**
   1. Procedure can be performed with moderate or minimal sedation.
F. **Intraprocedural care**
   1. Refer to Table 16.4 for intraprocedural care.

═══════════════════════════════*FAST FACTS in a NUTSHELL*

Ensure the foreign body is removed in its entirety, especially if it breaks during the procedure.

G. **Postprocedural care**
   1. Refer to Table 16.5 for basic postprocedural care.
H. **Complications**
   1. The most common complications associated with the procedure include infection, bleeding, and injury to the organs surrounding the foreign body.
I. **Follow-up/patient education**
   1. Patient follows up with primary care physician after procedure.
   2. Patient should contact primary care physician if puncture site demonstrates signs of infection, or if having swelling at puncture site, fever, or chills.

PART

V

# Diagnostic and Other Imaging Modalities

# 29

# X-Ray, Mammography, Nuclear Medicine, and Ultrasound

### Valerie Aarne Grossman

In this chapter, you will learn:

1. Patient preparation for exams
2. Necessary patient screening
3. Differences in imaging technology

All areas of the imaging environment pose a different set of challenges and expectations for the radiology nurse. Interventional radiology (IR), computed tomography (CT) scans, and magnetic resonance imaging (MRI) scans are the areas that utilize nursing personnel to the greatest degree; however, there are many other modalities within radiology that may, on occasion, also need the expertise of a nurse. The nurse who practices in a radiology setting must be ready to change direction at a moment's notice. Infinite reasons exist that may necessitate a radiologist, radiologic technologist, or a patient to call for a nurse (e.g., a patient may experience an adverse reaction to contrast or might require pain medicine during a routine exam).

# PROJECTION RADIOGRAPHY

## X-Ray

The use of radiation to capture images was first discovered in 1895 by a German physics professor and first used on patients in a clinical setting in 1896. The use of film and chemicals to develop the x-ray images has now been replaced by a digital process and computer screen. Plain x-rays remain the first-line image for many patient care situations.

## Fluoroscopy

This is a special application of x-ray imaging where real-time imaging is used to track motion. Often, contrast may be used to augment the image in the form of oral, rectal cavity, or intravenous contrast dye (see Chapter 9: CT Contrast Basics). The contrast will absorb the x-rays, highlight the motion process, and capture the images. This process is useful in assessing digestive tract peristalsis or blood flow through vessels.

Nursing interventions in this modality are often minimal to nothing at all. Radiologists and radiologic technologists provide the care for patients in this area (Ingles, Law, & Revell, 2010).

## Mammography

This low-dose radiographic technique has been practiced for more than 70 years to discover breast cysts or tumors. A *screening mammogram* is used to look for breast disease in asymptomatic women while a *diagnostic mammogram* is used to diagnose breast disease in symptomatic women or those with a finding during a screening mammogram. This new technology has many positive influences for both patients and staff that include the following:

- Easier for the patient
  - Decreases the need for additional images or return trips for additional films
- Decreases the amount of staff time to obtain/process images
- Increases the interpretation accuracy of the radiologist
  - Easy identification of dense versus nondense breast tissue and manipulation of images for more accurate interpretations

Nursing care in the mammography suite is minimal as the images are obtained by a radiologic technologist. Nurses may be utilized during adverse events or biopsy procedures.

## Patient Screening

The following indications for mammography should be considered:

- Annual exams for asymptomatic women age 40 and older who are at average risk for breast cancer
- Women under age 40 who are at increased risk for breast cancer
  - Known mutation or genetic syndrome with increased breast cancer risk starting annually between ages 25 and 30; that is, *BRCA1* or *BRCA2* mutation gene carriers
  - First-degree relative with known *BRCA* mutation, starting annually between ages 25 and 30
  - Sisters or mothers with premenopausal breast cancer, starting annually between the ages of 25 and 30 or 10 years earlier than the age of the relative's diagnosis
  - History of chest (mantle) radiation received between the ages of 10 and 30, starting annually 8 years after the radiation therapy, but not before age 25
  - Biopsy-proven lobular neoplasia, atypical ductal hyperplasia, ductal carcinoma in situ, invasive breast cancer, or ovarian cancer, starting annually from the time of diagnosis regardless of age (American College of Radiology, 2013a)
- Woman with breast augmentation
  - Must receive mammography services from a center equipped to image breasts with implants (Lee et al., 2010)

═══════════════════════════ *FAST FACTS in a NUTSHELL*

Proper patient preparation is essential to ensure a quality patient experience and perfection in the image quality of the exam.

## Patient Education

Patient education should begin when the appointment is first scheduled. The patient should be advised of the appropriate organization preparation requirements (i.e., insurance card, photo identification, avoid wearing deodorant/power/creams, and so on). The mammography technologist will continue the education by explaining the imaging procedure to the patient, answering her questions, helping to reduce the patient's anxiety, and instructing how the results will be handled.

## NUCLEAR MEDICINE

Images are obtained in this modality by injecting the patient with a radiopharmaceutical that locates to a particular type of body organ or tissue type and then imaging with a gamma camera. This is different from other imaging modalities as the radiation comes from the inside of the patient's body to the outside, where a camera obtains the image (other modalities direct the radiation from the camera through the body to obtain images). The most common images are obtained of the:

- Brain
- Heart, lungs
- Thyroid, parathyroid
- Bone
- Liver, gallbladder, spleen, or kidney
- Vessels that are causing internal bleeding
- Infection
- Collection of cells

Positron emission tomography is another imaging technique used in nuclear medicine, where a radioactive biological substance is injected into the patient and localizes to metabolically active tissues such as cancerous areas (Society of Nuclear Medicine and Molecular Imaging, 2013).

A nurse may be called to this area to perform point-of-care testing (POCT) for glucose, place an intravenous (IV) line, inject certain medication that may be used for scans, or respond to adverse patient events.

### Patient Screening

Patients will be screened for a medical history including allergies and pregnancy status.

Some patients will receive radioactive contrast and may need special documentation if they plan to travel through security checkpoints such as at an airport.

## Patient Education

Patient education should begin when the appointment is first scheduled. The patient should be advised per the organization's preparation policy (e.g., insurance card, photo identification, wearing comfortable clothing, nothing by mouth for certain exams, and so on). Upon the patient's arrival to the department, the nuclear medicine technologist will continue the educational process by explaining the imaging procedure, answering questions, and providing instruction regarding how test results can be obtained. This additional education helps to reduce the patient's anxiety.

## Ultrasound

This imaging technique uses high frequency sound waves to create the image that is interpreted by the radiologist. The first use of ultrasound occurred in the 1940s and has grown in use since then. Some important details to know about ultrasound:

- Ultrasound scan refers to the "procedure" of obtaining images
  - External: Probe placed outside of the body, looking inward
  - Internal: Probe placed inside the body
    - Vaginal internal probe to look at uterus and ovaries (women)
    - Rectal internal probe to look at the prostate gland (males)
  - Endoscopic: Probe placed through the mouth into the esophagus
    - Evaluates the esophagus, chest lymph nodes, or the stomach
- Sonogram is the actual image that is produced
- Doppler ultrasound images movement (e.g., blood flowing through a vessel)
  - Color may be used to identify flow patterns
- Ultrasound is useful in diagnostic imaging of the organs including:
  - Eye
  - Chest: Heart, vessels, lungs (images poorly through air; however, helpful when identifying fluid collection in the lungs)

- Abdomen: Stomach, liver
- Musculoskeletal: Tendons, muscles, joints
- Gastrointestinal/genitourinary/obstetrics: Scrotum, uterus
- Vascular: Blood vessels
- Therapeutic ultrasound is the use of sound waves to:
  - Cause coagulation necrosis of tissue
  - Stimulate bone growth
  - Help drugs pass the blood–brain barrier
  - Phacoemulsification of cataracts
  - Lithotripsy of kidney stones
- POCT ultrasound is a useful "bedside tool" in many areas—from the emergency department to the anesthesia department—to assist with patient assessment through initiation of care (e.g., IV line placement, bladder scanners, Doppler, and so on) (American College of Emergency Physicians, 2009).

For routine ultrasound exams, little nursing care is required. However, if a nurse is utilizing ultrasound to assist with IV cannulation, special training must occur prior to the use of ultrasound technology by that nurse. Additionally, if ultrasound is used during a procedure with a physician, the nurse may be administering pain medications and/or moderate sedation (see Chapter 6: Monitoring).

## Patient Screening

Ultrasound technology is highly dependent on the skill of the person using the equipment as well as the body habitus of the patient being examined (e.g., high quality images are difficult to obtain on very thin or obese patients). Minimal patient screening or preparation is needed prior to the use of ultrasound.

## Patient Education

Patient education should begin when the appointment is first scheduled. The patient should be advised per the organization's preparation policy (e.g., insurance card, photo identification, wearing comfortable clothing, nothing by mouth for certain exams, full bladder for other exams, and so on). The person performing the POCT ultrasound or the sonographer will continue the educational process by explaining the imaging procedure to the patient, answering questions, helping to reduce the patient's anxiety, and instructing how the results will be handled.

# Special Issues in Radiology Nursing

# 30

# Fragile and High-Risk Populations

## Valerie Aarne Grossman

In this chapter, you will learn:

1. The care of a pediatric patient
2. The care of a geriatric patient
3. Techniques in the care of high-risk/fragile patients

Radiology nursing is an exciting arena, as the nurse often doesn't know what is going to happen in the next few minutes—the variability of the patient population leaves a great deal unknown and unable to be planned for. Each patient brings unique identifiers that may add challenges to the nurse's goal of providing patient- and family-focused imaging care. It is essential for the nurse to recognize the unique needs of each individual patient and work to meet those needs with the ultimate outcome of quality patient care.

## PEDIATRIC

- The better the cooperation of the patient, the better the image obtained
- Educate the child (and guardian) prior to entering the modality if possible

- Use simple terms, just the basics; don't scare the child (or parent!)
- Advise of a big room, fancy camera, funny smells, weird noises, and so on
- Use terms understood by the child
- Never leave the child unattended
- When possible, allow the parent to remain in the room with the child
- Allow the child to bring a comfort item (toy, blanket, and so on)
- At times, sedation or immobilization (Velcro, tape, boards, and so on) may be utilized
- Use distraction when appropriate (visual, audio, personal interactions, and so on)
- Demonstrate using the parent ("Daddy is going to lay on the table first, then it's your turn")
- Protect the child from radiation exposure as much is possible

(Linder & Schiska, 2007; Matich, 2011; Munn & Jordan, 2013; Reilly, Byrne, & Ely, 2012)

## FAST FACTS in a NUTSHELL

Taking the time to include the parent/caregiver in the care of the child will help the child to become more comfortable in the strange environment of any radiology setting. Making the exam seem like "play" will allow for better image quality and decrease the potential traumatic experience for the child.

## GERIATRIC

- Identify communication barriers and find solutions (hearing impaired, slow speech pattern, slow cognition, and so on)
- Physical barriers such as decreased strength, slower walking, unsteady gait, easily fatigued, diminished eyesight, and so on
- Careful patient assessment for history, current medications, and so on
- Fragile; easy skin tearing, difficult intravenous cannulation, easy bruising
- Foster autonomy wherever possible, communicate on the patient's level
- Provide for physical comfort (padding, wedges, blankets, and so on)

# CHEMICALLY ALTERED PATIENTS

- Patients who have received pain medication or sedation prior to coming to radiology may easily fall, have decreased ability to cooperate with directions, may easily forget instructions, and so on
- Patients who have consumed mind-altering chemicals may be uncooperative and at times, a danger to the radiology staff. Monitor them closely; utilize security if necessary

# MORBIDLY OBESE

- Be open, honest, and nonjudgmental with larger patients if there are concerns regarding their care due to their size
- Obtain a current and accurate weight on the patient; do NOT use the stated weight
- Verify table weight limit prior to placing the patient on the table
- Educate the patient regarding the use of wedges, belts, and other safety devices used to maintain proper patient position during exam
- Contrast may be weight based; be careful of dose limits
- Measure patient girth to be sure the patient will fit in scanner gantries/apertures (Grossman, 2009)

# COGNITIVE DISORDERS

- Identify the ability of the patient to comprehend instructions
- Speak at a level understood by the patient/family

# EXTREME STRESS OR FEAR

- It is imperative for staff to recognize the anxiety level of the patient
- Work to provide a confident and calm environment for the patient/family
- Fear of the unknown is powerful, so work to educate the patient from the very first interaction

Honest communication with all patients will promote a smoother experience for the patient. The radiology environment is "strange and unknown" for most patients.

## CULTURALLY DIVERSE

- Different groups may perceive a situation differently
  - The nurse may not understand the background of each patient; however, the nurse can be sensitive to the fears a patient may have from not understanding the technical radiology setting
- Work to find a common ground of understanding; use interpreters, listen for concerns, take time to teach and answer questions, provide for patient comfort, and so forth
- Portray confidence, acceptance, patience, and friendliness to all patients
- Identify own biases or prejudices, and work to keep them out of the workplace (Grossman, 2003; Jan & Nardi, 2005)

# 31

# Current Trends in Nursing Care

## Polly Gerber Zimmermann

In this chapter, you will discover:

1. New twists to old skills
2. Updated nursing basics
3. Updated safety actions

Depending on how "seasoned" a nurse is, the memory trail of past or outdated practices can be quite long. There are social/environmental changes such as nursing caps. More important are quality and safety advances in providing health care. Who can remember the days of:

- Caregiving without gloves (it would offend the patient)
- Milking chest tubes
- Humidifiers with standing water in patients' rooms
- Venous cutdowns (instead of PICC or peripherally inserted central catheter lines)
- Checking a patient's glucose level with tablets and urine in a test tube instead of using blood

Some more recent nursing evolutions include the following practices.

# LOCATION OF INTRAMUSCULAR INJECTIONS

- Intramuscular injections larger than 1 mL (for those aged 7 months or older) are given in the ventrogluteal area (gluteus medius, anterior gluteal site), not the dorsogluteal (butt, upper outer quadrant, gluteus maximus).
- Even a properly located dorsogluteal injection still has the risk of nerve or artery injury.
- The ventrogluteal site has no major complications ever attributed to it because it avoids all major nerves and blood vessels.
- In addition, the body's fat is more evenly distributed making it a shorter distance to reach the muscle (Zimmermann, 2010).

## Procedure to Locate Ventrogluteal Area

Palpate the greater trochanter (feels like a golf ball).

- Place the palm of your hand on top of the trochanter.
- Position the index finger on or pointing toward the anterior superior iliac spine.
- Spread apart the third finger from the index finger.
- Administer the injection in the center of the "V" or triangle formed by the two fingers.

### Hints for the best intramuscular (IM) injection technique include:

- Positioning the patient either in the Sim's position (side-lying patient with top leg in front of bottom leg with knee bent) or prone with the toes pointed inward
- Applying manual pressure firmly for 10 seconds before inserting the needle. (It stimulates the surrounding nerve endings.)
- Inserting the needle at a 90° insertion angle
- Stretching, rather than pinching, the skin (unless emaciated)
- Using Z-track technique (displacing the skin by 2.5 to 3.75 cm laterally before puncturing it, releasing as withdrawing the needle to "seal off" the site).

- Depressing the plunger slowly at a rate of 10 seconds per mL to allow the fluid to absorb.
- Unless the dorsogluteal is used, there is no need to aspirate for *any* injection.

## Foley Urinary Catheters

It is no longer recommended that the Foley urinary catheter balloon be tested prior to insertion as it has been tested in the factory. The risk is that the balloon won't be completely deflated before insertion. To aid insertion in a male, use the provided lubrication in the syringe instilled directly into the meatus for dilation.

The old wisdom was to clamp a Foley catheter after insertion if the output reached 1,000 mL. The thought was to prevent shock from losing too much volume too quickly in a patient with bladder distention. Now it is considered safe to allow the entire bladder amount to come out immediately upon installation of the catheter.

## Glucose Control

Insulin management is moving toward the routine use of a steady-level basal insulin (glargine, Lantus) supplemented with a rapid acting insulin that takes effect almost immediately (Novolog, Aspart, Lispro).

Type 2 diabetes is now recognized as having issues not only with insulin deficiency, but insulin resistance, increased hepatic glucose release, and impaired glucose storage. Type 2 tends to be progressive, eventually requiring a second oral drug or insulin (40% of type 2 diabetics will eventually require insulin).

- The new emphasis is for tight glucose control below 150 mg as hyperglycemia affects morbidity.
- Sliding scale coverage for hyperglycemia is considered less effective than an insulin drip, as you are always "behind."
- Acute hypoglycemia in the semiconscious patient often is treated initially with only 25 mL of 50% dextrose (instead of the entire vial) to prevent rebound hypoglycemia.
  - Administer glucagon 1 mg IM if intravenous (IV) access is not readily available.

> Position the patient to avoid aspiration as vomiting is common following the administration of glucagon.

## INTRAOSSEOUS ACCESS DEVICES

Intraosseous (IO) access provides access to the noncollapsible venous plexus in the bone marrow space, thus enabling drug delivery similar to that achieved by central venous access. IO cannulation is now appropriate for settings when IV access cannot be obtained and the patient would be compromised without the medication or solutions that have been prescribed for an emergent clinical condition (including rapid response team algorithms). There is limited information, but a case study and animal studies indicate that the IO site can be used for IV contrast dye in adults if there is no IV access available. Concerns still exist if a power rate injection should be used.

The Infusion Nurses Society (INS) Position Paper indicates a qualified registered nurse (RN) may insert, maintain, and remove IO access devices. The RN (depending on the state's Nurse Practice Act) must be:

- Proficient in infusion therapy
- Appropriately trained for the procedure (Consortium on Intraosseous Vascular Access in Healthcare Practice, 2010)

## MAGNESIUM MATTERS

Consider magnesium levels when potassium, another intracellular electrolyte, is subtherapeutic. Adequate magnesium is essential to be able to utilize the administered potassium.

## ALCOHOLISM/ALCOHOL WITHDRAWAL

Approximately 18 million people in the United States have an alcohol use disorder. Monitor admitted patients, especially those who had an unplanned admission (such as through the emergency department), for potential alcohol withdrawal. The onset for delirium tremens (DTs) is 6 to 8 hours after the last drink. Alcohol withdrawal seizures can occur 6 to 96 hours *after* the last drink. Use the Clinical Institute Withdrawal Assessment for Alcohol, Revised (CTWA-Ar). Items assessed include nausea/vomiting; tremor; paroxysmal sweats; tactile, auditory, or visual disturbances; anxiety; headache; agitation; and orientation. Consider the risk of alcohol-induced hypoglycemia (AIH) from insufficient glycogen stores and the alcohol-induced impairment of gluconeogenesis. It occurs during intoxication or up to 20 hours after the last drink (NIAAA, 2013).

━━━━━━━━━━━━━━━━━━━━━*FAST FACTS in a NUTSHELL*

Patients at risk for AIH are chronic alcoholics, binge drinkers, and young children.

## DELIRIUM VERSUS DEMENTIA

Dementia is a slow, progressive worsening of cognition/memory and at least one other feature, but an alert mental status. Delirium is a symptom of another problem with an alteration in alertness (hypoactive, hyperactive or fluctuating).

Triggers can include:

- Worsening infection
- Fluid and electrolyte imbalance
- New medication (especially a psychotropic)

Use the short Confusion Assessment Method (CAM). The patient must have 1, 2, and 3 or 4.

- A mental status altered from the baseline AND
- Inattention (easily distracted, unable to spell "world" backwards) AND
- Disorganized thinking (rambling, illogical, hallucinations) OR
- Altered level of consciousness (anything but alert) (Waszynski, 2007).

# 32

# Communication Essentials Between the Emergency Department and Radiology

## Anna C. Montejano and Lynn Sayre Visser

In this chapter, you will discover:

1. The value of a safe hand-off
2. Essentials of coordination of care
3. Patient preparation for transport

Communication between the emergency department (ED) and the radiology staff is of high importance to ensure patient safety because:

- When vital information is not communicated among staff, a patient may be at risk for injury.
- Communication also plays a role in knowing when both the ED and radiology staff are ready for the patient to be transported to radiology.
- Communication between departments is essential in understanding when and why delays occur and provides a smooth transition between care providers.

# WHEN RADIOLOGY IS READY FOR THE ED PATIENT

Both radiology and emergency are very busy departments. Coordination of schedules must occur to optimize smooth progress in the care of the mutual patient. Communication by telephone between the radiology staff and the primary registered nurse (RN) prior to patient transport from ED to radiology enhances departmental efficiency and improves patient care.

## PREPARING THE ED PATIENT FOR RADIOLOGY

The ED nurse should be informed prior to the patient being transported to radiology as:

- Certain procedures may require the paper chart to accompany the patient and valuable time can be saved if this is identified during patient preparation for transport.
- Oxygen may be needed for the transport of some patients to radiology.

## *FAST FACTS in a NUTSHELL*

Be sure the oxygen tank used for transport has enough oxygen to support the needs of the patient (a higher flow may require a full tank while a lower flow rate may only require a minimum of 500 psi).

- Testing such as blood work, an electrocardiogram (ECG), and other diagnostic tests may be required prior to the radiologic procedure or exam.
- Intravenous (IV) access may be required: Assess the catheter size and placement location most appropriate for the total care of the patient.
- If the patient is receiving a fluid bolus, the nurse may need to slow down the fluid or hang another IV bag prior to the transport to radiology.
- The patient may require medication prior to transfer to radiology to control nausea, provide pain relief, or begin combatting an infectious process with antibiotics.

- If the ED is waiting for a urine sample from the patient, this information should be communicated to the radiology staff prior to patient transport to radiology.
- Valuables including necklaces, earrings, nipple or belly button rings, dentures, or hearing aids may need to be removed prior to obtaining films.
- Acutely ill patients may need a nurse to accompany them to radiology to provide continuous assessment and evaluate cardiac monitoring, respiratory effort, and medication needs.

========================*FAST FACTS in a NUTSHELL*

ED patients often require a multitude of orders that must be carried out in addition to the radiology test. ED staff must prioritize the needed tests and communicate clearly to the radiology staff as to when the patient is ready to be transported

## UPON TRANSPORT TO RADIOLOGY— TICKET TO RIDE

The Joint Commission (TJC) International Patient Safety Goal No. 2 focuses on enhancing communication (World Health Organization [WHO], 2007). Between 1995 and 2006, reports to TJC confirmed insufficient communication as the primary cause of sentinel events (The Joint Commission Center for Transforming Healthcare, 2013). As a result of these reports, the Ticket to Ride was developed as one avenue for standardizing communication among staff and to support improved patient safety. Depending on the organization's process, there may be a combination of paper and electronic methods for this communication process. Components for the Ticket to Ride should include the following:

- Placing the Ticket to Ride on colored paper for easy visualization.
- Developing the tool in a Situation/Background/Assessment/ Recommendation (SBAR) format to ensure a thorough and standardized form of communication (WHO, 2007).
  - *Situation* includes the imaging studies ordered for the patient (e.g., CT) and the reason for the procedure (e.g., chest x-ray to rule out pneumonia). Verification that

the patient is wearing an identification bracelet with an accurate date of birth and correct spelling of the name is critical.

- *Background* provides information regarding the patient's diagnosis, code status, and orientation. Additionally, fall risk, ability to stand, isolation, communication (native language), do not resuscitate (DNR) status, and deficits in hearing or vision are identified.
- *Assessment* includes the patient's current condition. Invaluable information to report to transporting staff includes the presence of IV lines, tubes, or drains, oxygen needs, or sedating medications given.
- *Recommendation* includes providing a phone number in the ED to call for questions as well as the patient's primary nurse/physician.

## PATIENT'S RETURN TO THE ED FROM RADIOLOGY

It is essential for the nurse to know when the patient returns to the ED:

- The nurse can gauge the timeline of anticipated radiology reports.
- Verbal patient hand-off supports best practice.
- Wall oxygen may need to be resumed before the oxygen tank potentially becomes empty.
- Cardiac monitoring may need to be continued in the ED.
- Diagnostic testing that was not initiated prior to transport needs to be completed.
- Possible reaction to contrast needs to be monitored by the ED RN in case interventions are needed (e.g., rash requiring diphenhydramine).

## FAST FACTS in a NUTSHELL

Communication with the ED nurse that the patient has returned to the ED supports best practice in patient hand-off, enhancing patient safety and yielding opportunity for the delivery of timely continued care.

A number of reasons exist requiring the ED staff to delay transport to radiology. The ED RN and physician, as well as the radiology staff, must continuously prioritize care of all patients.

Reasons for delay include:

- The ED radiology patient is bumped by a patient presenting with a more acute presentation within the hospital or ED.
- Procedures and/or tests that require completion prior to the radiologic exam:
  - A septic patient requires a series of tests to be performed within a designated time frame (e.g., lactate level, blood cultures, antibiotics, and fluid).
  - Nausea or pain. Controlling patient nausea or pain prior to transport enhances patient comfort, improves patient cooperation, and increases efficiency for radiology staff.
- Oral contrast: The patient may not have consumed the required volume of contrast due to the patient sleeping, nausea, vomiting, or pain.
- IV access: The nurse may face difficulty obtaining appropriate IV access suitable for IV contrast.
- Test results: ED staff maybe waiting for results to be reported so the ordered diagnostic exam can be completed (e.g., creatinine, urine pregnancy test, beta HCG).

## FAST FACTS in a NUTSHELL

Communication between ED and radiology staff is critical to quality patient care. Staff experience high levels of frustration when insufficient communication occurs. Taking time to communicate enhances work efficiency for staff and improves patient outcomes.

# 33

# Preparing Emergency Department Patients for Radiologic Procedures

## Lynn Sayre Visser and Anna C. Montejano

In this chapter, you will discover:

1. The importance of timing and communication
2. Core measures
3. Patient preparation for imaging

Twenty-four hours a day, 7 days a week, 365 days a year, emergency department (ED) staff stand ready to provide each arriving patient with quality care. Some patient presentations require rapid treatment and intervention, while other presentations are less acute. Patients sometimes arrive to the ED with vague complaints, thus uncovering the covert clues that lead to a timely and accurate medical diagnosis is essential. Although in many facilities the ED and radiology departments are separate entities, both departments are vital to the patient experience and the outcome.

# CORE MEASURES

*Core measure* is a national initiative used to determine the quality of hospital performance and patient care. Acute myocardial infarction (AMI), pneumonia, and stroke are the most common core measure presentations seen in the ED. Nurses play a key role with core measures by organizing the necessary collaboration of hospital staff. The radiology staff play an important role in meeting core measures.

## Acute Myocardial Infarction

- The ECG should be completed within 10 minutes and shown to an ED physician for interpretation (Antman et al., 2004).
- A thrombolytic must be administered within 30 minutes from the time of patient arrival in the ED (Antman et al., 2004).
- Prior to administering a thrombolytic (e.g., tissue plasminogen activator, streptokinase), a chest x-ray (CXR) must be completed to rule out an aortic aneurysm.
  - When a cardiac catheterization suite is available and the procedure is deemed appropriate for the patient, the timeline from door to percutaneous coronary intervention is 90 minutes (Antman et al., 2004).

## Pneumonia

- A patient who arrives with symptoms of pneumonia needs a CXR as soon as possible so that the pneumonia core measure can be implemented.
- Timely antibiotic administration is the essential component of this core measure.
- The goal for door to antibiotic time is less than 4 hours.
- Prior to the administration of antibiotic, two sets of blood cultures should be obtained.

## Stroke

- A patient who exhibits signs and symptoms of a stroke will need a rapid CT of the head (to determine the type of stroke—hemorrhagic or ischemic) within established time frames from the National Institutes of Neurological Disorders and Stroke (NINDS):

- CT should be completed 25 minutes or less from the time of arrival to the ED.
- CT should be interpreted by a radiologist within 40 minutes from the time the patient arrives in the ED.
- Rapid availability of the CT scanner, radiology staff, and a radiologist is imperative.
- Identification of stroke patients focuses on the time the patient was last seen normal with a 3-hour time limit for a patient to receive thrombolytic therapy (Jauch et al., 2013).

==== *FAST FACTS in a NUTSHELL*

- Meeting the timelines with 100% efficiency not only provides quality evidence-based care and patient safety, but shows the ability of the hospital to follow requirements developed by The Joint Commission and the Centers of Medicare & Medicaid Services.
- ED staff frequently reference core measure order sets to ensure completion of the essential core measure criteria.
- Always remember that we all play a role in core measures. Efficient intradepartmental teamwork and communication results in high-quality patient care.

## COMMON ED RADIOLOGICAL PROCEDURES

### X-Ray

- Depending on the acuity of the patient presentation, x-rays may be ordered in a portable mode or the patient may go to the radiology department.
- Portable films may be essential when:
  - The patient is too unstable for transfer to the radiology department.
  - A patient is in moderate/severe respiratory distress requiring simultaneous nebulizer treatments and intravenous medications.

- Confirmation of the endotracheal tube placement is required.
- Confirmation of a central line placement is required.
- Postprocedural monitoring (e.g., hip or shoulder dislocation) is necessary.
- Core measure treatments require multiple tests to occur simultaneously.
- Prior to obtaining a portable film there are several considerations including:
  - Positioning for a portable CXR requires careful consideration of the medical condition and communication with the ED staff.
  - Conditions such as hypotension or a labile head injury may not allow the patient to sit upright.
  - Intubated patients require precautions to protect the airway during any x-ray.
  - Restrained patients need staff to be cognizant of harm risk when restraints are loosened.
  - When placing the film behind the patient, staff must be vigilant not to disconnect intravenous lines, Foley catheters, nasogastric tubes, and so on.

## *FAST FACTS in a NUTSHELL*

X-rays provide valuable information to ED staff. A quick response time on radiology reads for postintubation and postline placement films is imperative so that necessary treatment can be initiated and/or continued. Adverse outcomes from the procedure can be ruled out and potentially vital treatment can be initiated once placement is confirmed.

## Magnetic Resonance Imaging (MRI)

- Patient screening prior to an MRI for the possibility of internal metal objects, pain, claustrophobia, contrast allergy, and so on, often occurs in the ED prior to the transfer to MRI.
  - The ED nurse may administer ordered medication to ensure pain management, control of anxiety, adequate sedation, or contrast allergy premedication.

## Computed Tomography (CT)

- CT scans are a common diagnostic procedure for the ED patient as they provide a quick and complete report of internal function and dysfunction.
  - Prioritization of patients in the CT queue is essential so that the potentially sickest patients are treated first (trauma, stroke, pulmonary embolism, and so on).

## Ultrasound

- Often used to rapidly assess the possibility of a testicular torsion or ectopic pregnancy.
  - Some special patient preparation may be required, such as placement of a Foley catheter and/or the patient having a full bladder.

## PATIENT SAFETY IS FIRST . . . ALWAYS

Following any radiological test or procedure, always think about patient safety. If side rails were lowered or the height of the gurney was raised to complete the radiological order, place the side rails back up and leave the patient's gurney in a low position. If the patient's status changes in any way during the procedure, the ED nurse or physician must be notified so an assessment and appropriate follow-up care can be provided.

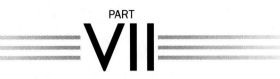

PART

# VII

# Emerging Areas of Radiology Nursing

# 34

## Orientation, Certification, and Point-of-Care Testing

### Valerie Aarne Grossman

In this chapter, you will discover:

1. The importance of proper job orientation
2. Point-of-care testing (POCT) for the radiology nurse
3. Certification in radiology nursing

## NURSING ORIENTATION

The orientation to the radiology environment for each new nurse will be developed based on the services provided and the patient population of the organization. Because the role of a radiology nurse is independent, many departments will recruit nurses with solid experience in critical care. Radiology nurses must have an expert command of patient care under difficult circumstances (patient acuity, fast paced, different sets of information to synthesize, all age groups, and so on). To have a successful orientation program, each department should have:

- Strong leadership with clear team goals (Aarne Grossman, 2013a)
- Skilled preceptors with sincere passion for mentoring

- Well-defined orientation objectives for each modality to which the nurse may be called
- Ample training for each modality
  - May need 160 to 320 hours of orientation for interventional radiology (IR) procedures
  - May need 40 hours of orientation for individual modalities (i.e., CT, MRI, and so on).
- Checklists and competency documentation of stated orientation objectives
- Registration in hospital-offered classes (i.e., advanced cardiac life support [ACLS], telemetry, critical care, and so on).
- Weekly meetings with manager, preceptor, and orientee to discuss successes and hurdles of orientation progression
- Post orientation evaluation (Sousa, 2013)

## FAST FACTS in a NUTSHELL

Due to changes in health care funding, many organizations are shortening the length of nursing orientation. Make careful choices when planning the education of your new staff: the investment YOU make in your orientation program will ultimately provide your patients with a safer and higher quality experience.

## CERTIFICATION IN RADIOLOGY NURSING

A goal for all radiology nurses should be membership in the Association for Radiologic & Imaging Nursing as well as certification in their specialty. To be eligible to take the certification exam in radiology nursing, a nurse must:

- Possess a current and active registered nurse license in his or her state or the international licensure equivalent
- Have practiced in the radiology setting for a minimum of 2,000 hours in the previous 3 years
- Obtained 30 contact hours of approved continuing education within the previous 24 months, with a minimum of 15 hours specifically related to radiology nursing

Once obtained, certification is valid for 4 years from the date of passing the exam.

Bedside testing has changed over the past decade, and in many states may be heavily regulated. The radiology nurse may need to be proficient in the following POCT techniques:

- Blood glucose
- Urine pregnancy
- Serum creatinine, blood urea nitrogen, estimated glomerular filtration rate for contrast decisions
- Handheld Doppler for checking pulses
- Handheld ultrasound for IV placement
- Activated clotting time (for interventional radiology procedural care)

The nurse will be required to follow the guidelines as established by governing agencies and organizational policy.

════════════════════════════════════*FAST FACTS in a NUTSHELL*

Point-of-care testing is an important enhancement of patient care that occurs in the image and procedural settings. Regulations regarding its use are often complicated; however, the effort is essential for our practice areas.

# Abbreviations

| | |
|---|---|
| ABHR | Alcohol-based hand rub |
| ACA | Affordable Care Act |
| ACEP | American College of Emergency Physicians (www.acep.org) |
| ACLS | Advanced Cardiac Life Support course |
| ACR | American College of Radiology (www.acr.org) |
| ACT | Activated clotting time |
| ACTH | Adrenocorticotropic hormone |
| ADH | Atypical ductal hyperplasia |
| AHRQ | Agency for Healthcare Research and Quality (Department of Health and Human Services) (www.ahrq.gov) |
| AIH | Alcohol-induced hypoglycemia |
| AMI | Acute myocardial infarction |
| AORN | Association of periOperative Registered Nurses (www.aorn.org) |
| ARIN | Association for Radiologic & Imaging Nursing (www.arinursing.org) |
| ARRA | American Recovery and Reinvestment Act of 2009 (www.recovery.gov) |
| aPTT | Activated partial thromboplastin time |
| ASA | American Society of Anesthesiologists |
| AVF | Arterial venous fistula |
| AVJ | Atrioventricular junction |

| AVM | Arteriovenous malformation |
|---|---|
| BOH | Bundle of His |
| BPA | Best practice advisory |
| *BRCA1* | Human gene |
| *BRCA2* | Human gene |
| BUN | Blood urea nitrogen |
| CAD | Coronary artery disease |
| CAT Scan | Computerized axial tomography scan |
| C-Diff | *Clostridium difficile* |
| CDC | Centers for Disease Control and Prevention (www.cdc.gov) |
| CHF | Congestive heart failure |
| CIRA | Canadian Interventional Radiology Association (www.ciraweb.org) |
| CIRSE | Cardiovascular and Interventional Radiology Society of Europe (www.cirse.org) |
| CMS | Centers for Medicaid & Medicare Services (www.cms.gov) |
| COPD | Chronic obstructed pulmonary disease |
| CRE | Carbapenem-resistant *Enterobacteriaceae* |
| CRH | Corticotropin-releasing hormone |
| CSF | Cerebral spinal fluid |
| CT | Computed tomography |
| CTWA-Ar | Clinical Institute Withdrawal Assessment for Alcohol, Revised |
| CVC | Central venous catheter |
| CXR | Chest x-ray |
| DCIS | Ductal carcinoma in situ (breast cancer) |
| DICOM | Digital Imaging and Communications in Medicine |
| DDAVP | 1-deamino-8-D-arginine vasopressin |
| DNR | Do not resuscitate |
| DT | Delirium tremens |
| DVT | Deep vein thrombosis |
| ECG | Electrocardiogram |
| ED ("ER") | Emergency department (emergency room) |
| eGFR | Estimated glomerular filtration rate |

| eHR | Electronic health record |
|---|---|
| EMR | Electronic medical record |
| ENA | Emergency Nurses Association (www.ena.org) |
| ESBL | Extended-spectrum beta-lactamase–producing organisms |
| ESRD | End-stage renal disease |
| ETT | Endotracheal tube |
| EVLA | Endovenous laser ablation |
| FDA | U.S Food and Drug Administration (www.fda.gov) |
| FFP | Fresh frozen plasma |
| GSV | Greater saphenous vein |
| GI | Gastrointestinal |
| GU | Genitourinary |
| HBV | Hepatitis B virus |
| HCG | Human chorionic gonadotropin |
| HCV | Hepatitis C virus |
| HIPAA | Health Insurance Portability and Accountability Act of 1996 (HIPAA) (www.hipaasurvivalguide.com/hipaa-regulations/hipaa-regulations.php) |
| HITECH | Health Information Technology for Economic and Clinical Health (www.hipaasurvivalguide.com/hitech-act-text.php) |
| HOB | Head of bed |
| HOPPS | Hospital Outpatient Perspective Payment System (www.cms.gov/Outreach-and-Education/Medicare-Learning-Network-MLN/MLNProducts/downloads/hospitaloutpaysysfctsht.pdf) |
| HTN | Hypertension |
| IA | Intra-arterial |
| ICP | Intracranial pressure |
| ICU | Intensive care unit |
| INR | International normalized ratio |
| INS | Infusion Nurses Society (www.ins1.org) |
| IO | Intraosseous (vascular access) |
| IR | Interventional radiology |

| | |
|---|---|
| IVC | Inferior vena cava |
| KDOQI | Kidney Disease Outcome Quality Initiative (www.kidney.org/professionals/kdoqi/index.cfm) |
| LDH | Lactate dehydrogenase |
| LOC | Level of consciousness |
| LSV | Lesser saphenous vein |
| LVAD | Left ventricular assist device |
| MAR | Medication administration record |
| MDR-GNB | Multidrug-resistant gram-negative bacteria |
| MI | Myocardial infarction |
| mL | Milliliter |
| mmHg | Millimeter(s) of mercury |
| MRA | Magnetic resonance angiography |
| MRI | Magnetic resonance imaging |
| MRSA | Methicillin-resistant *Staphylococcus aureus* |
| NaCL | Sodium chloride |
| nBCA | n-Butyl cyanoacrylate |
| NIH | National Institutes of Health (www.nih.gov) |
| NINDS | National Institutes of Neurological Disorders and Stroke |
| NKF | National Kidney Foundation (www.kidney.org) |
| NPO | Nil per os (nothing by mouth) |
| NSAID | Nonsteroidal anti-inflammatory drug |
| NSR | Normal sinus rhythm |
| OB | Obstetric |
| OR | Operating room |
| OSHA | Occupational Safety and Health Administration (www.osha.gov) |
| PACS | Picture archiving and communication system |
| PAD | Peripheral arterial disease |
| PAVM | Pulmonary arteriovenous malformations |
| PCA | Patient-controlled analgesia |
| PE | Pulmonary embolus |
| PEA | Pulseless electrical activity |
| PET scan | Positron emission tomography |

| PICC | Peripherally inserted central catheter |
| PIV | Peripheral intravenous catheter |
| POCT | Point-of-care testing |
| PPE | Personal protective equipment |
| PRBC | Packed red blood cells |
| PSA | Procedural sedation and analgesia |
| PSI | Pounds per square inch |
| PT | Prothrombin time |
| PTC | Percutaneous transhepatic cholangiography |
| PTT | Partial thromboplastin time |
| RIS | Radiology information system |
| RN | Registered nurse |
| RRS | Rapid response system |
| SAH | Subarachnoid hemorrhage |
| SA node | Sinoatrial node |
| SIIM | Society for Imaging Informatics in Medicine (www.siimweb.org) |
| SIR | Society of Interventional Radiology (www.sirweb.org) |
| SNMMI | Society of Nuclear Medicine and Molecular Imaging (interactive.snm.org/index.cfm?PageID=1176) |
| SPECT | Single photon emission computed tomography imaging |
| SSI | Surgical site infection |
| STAT | Immediate |
| STEM | Situation, treatment, event, meds |
| SVC | Superior vena cava |
| TACE | Transcatheter arterial chemoembolization |
| TB | Tuberculosis |
| TCVC | Tunneled cuffed venous catheters |
| TIPSS | Transjugular intrahepatic portosystemic shunt |
| tPA | Tissue plasminogen activator |
| UIP | Union Internationale de Phlebologie |
| VRE | Vancomycin-resistant enterococci |

# Bibliography

Aarne Grossman, V. (2013a). Hot topics: CT contrast and intraosseous lines: Friends or enemies? *Journal of Radiology Nursing, 31*(1), 41–44.

Aarne Grossman, V. (2013b). Teamwork essentials: Success in the radiology environment. *Journal of Radiology Nursing, 32*(3), 139–140.

American College of Emergency Physicians. (2009). Policy statement: Emergency ultrasound guidelines. *Annals of Emergency Medicine, 53,* 550–570.

American College of Radiology. (2013a). *ACR practice guideline for the performance of screening and diagnostic mammography.* Retrieved from www.acr.org/~/media/ACR/Documents/PGTS/guidelines/Screening_Mammography.pdf

American College of Radiology. (2013b). *Manual on contrast media, version 9.* Retrieved from www.acr.org/Quality-Safety/Resources/Contrast-Manual

American Heart Association. (2012). *Stroke fact sheet.* Retrieved from www.heart.org. doi:10.1161/01.CIR.0000134791.68010.FA

American Society of Anesthesiologists Task Force on Sedation and Analgesia by Non-anesthesiologists. (2002). Practice guidelines for sedation and analgesia by non-anesthesiologists. *Anesthesiology, 96*(4), 1004–1117.

Antman, E. M., Anbe, D. T., Armstrong, P. W., Bates, E. R., Green, L. A., Hand, M., . . . Jacobs, A. K. (2004). ACC/AHA guidelines for the management of patients with ST-elevation myocardial infarction—Executive summary: A report of the American College of Cardiology/American Heart Association Task Force on Practice Guidelines. *Circulation, 110,* 588–636.

Association of periOperative Registered Nurses. (2012). Recommended practices for prevention of transmissible infections in the perioperative setting. In *Perioperative standards and recommended practices* (pp. e91–e123). Denver, CO: Author. Retrieved from www.guideline.gov/content.aspx?id=43785

Association of periOperative Registered Nurses, Corner, R., & Blanchard, J. C. (2011). *Perioperative standards and recommended practices*. Denver, CO: Association of periOperative Registered Nurses.

Barker, E. (2008). *Neuroscience nursing: A spectrum of care* (3rd ed.). St. Louis, MO: Mosby.

Beckmann, E. (2006). CT scanning in the early days. *British Journal of Radiology, 79*, 5–8.

Bessell-Browne, R., & O'Malley, M. E. (2007). CT of pheochromocytoma and paraganglioma: Risk of adverse events with IV administration of nonionic contrast material. *American Journal of Roentgenology, 188*(4), 970–974.

Bratzler, D., Dellinger, E., Olsen, K., Perl, T., Auwaerter, P., Bolon, M., . . . Weinstein, R. (2013). Clinical practice guidelines for antimicrobial prophylaxis in surgery. *American Society of Health-System Pharmacists, 70*(3), 195–283. doi:10.2146/ajhp120568

Brenner, D. J. (2012). Minimising medically unwarranted computed tomography scans. *Annals of the International Commission on Radiological Protection, 41*(3–4), 161–169. doi:10.1016/j.icrp.2012.06.004

Brown, M., Mattrey, R., Stamato, S., & Sirlin, C. (2005). MRI of the female pelvis using vaginal gel. *American Journal of Roentgenology, 185*(5), 1221–1227.

Brunberg, J. A., Frey, K. A., Horton, J. A., Deveikis, J. P., Ross, D. A., & Koeppe, R. A. (1994). Positron emission tomography determination of cerebral blood flow during balloon test occlusion of the internal carotid artery. *AJNR. American Journal of Neuroradiology, 15*, 725–732.

Cammermeyer, M., & Appeldorn, C. (2010). *Core curriculum for neuroscience nursing* (5th ed.). Chicago, IL: American Association of Neuroscience Nurses.

Carroll, R., & Matfin, G. (2010). Endocrine and metabolic emergencies: Thyroid storm. *Therapeutic Advances in Endocrinology and Metabolism, 1*(3), 139–145.

Chan, D., Downing, D., Keough, C., Saad, W., & Annamalai, G. (2012). Joint practice guideline for sterile technique during vascular and interventional radiology procedures: From the Society of Interventional Radiology, Association of periOperative Registered Nurses, and Association for Radiologic and Imaging Nursing, for the Society of Interventional Radiology (Wael Saad, MD, Chair), Standards of Practice Committee, and endorsed by the Cardiovascular Interventional Radiological Society of Europe and the Canadian Interventional Radiology Association. *The Journal of Radiology Nursing, 31*(4), 130–143.

Consortium on Intraosseous Vascular Access in Healthcare Practice. (2010). *Recommendations for the use of intraosseous vascular access for emergent and nonemergent situations in various healthcare settings: A consensus paper.* Retrieved from www.ins1 .org/i4a/pages/index.cfm?pageid=3412

Cunha, B. (2013). *Antibiotic essentials.* Burlington, MA: Jones and Bartlett Learning.

Donnelly, L., Dickerson, J., Goodfriend, M., & Muething, S. (2010). Improving patient safety in radiology. *American Journal of Roentgenology, 194,* 1183–1187.

Glorsky, S., Wonderlich, D., & Goei, A. (2010). Evaluation and management of the trauma patient for the interventional radiologist. *Seminars in Interventional Radiology, 27*(1), 29–37.

Greenberg, D., & Scovell, S. (2012, June 26). *Liquid and foam sclerotherapy techniques for the treatment of lower extremity veins.* Retrieved from http://www.uptodate.com/contents/search

Grossman, V. A. (2003). Cross cultural empathy. In *Quick reference to triage.* Philadelphia, PA: Lippincott, Williams, & Wilkins.

Grossman, V. A. (2009). Imaging tips for overweight and obese patients. *RN Magazine/Modern Medicine.* Retrieved from www .modernmedicine.com

Grossman, V. A. (2012). Hot topics: Safe CT power injections of central venous catheters. *Journal of Radiology Nursing, 31*(3), 105–107.

Harrigan, M. R., & Deveikis, J. P. (2013). *Handbook of cerebrovascular disease and neurointerventional technique.* New York, NY: Springer.

Health Information Technology. (2013). Retrieved from www .healthit.gov

Health Protection Agency/Public Health England. (2011). *Press release: Scale of UK exposure to X-rays revealed.* Retrieved from www .hpa.org.uk/NewsCentre/NationalPressReleases/2011Press Releases/110104scaleofxrayexposurerevealed

Ihnat, D. (2012, September 11). Endovenous laser ablation for the treatment of lower extremity chronic venous disease. *Uptodate .com.*

Infusion Nurses Society. (2008). *Position paper: The role of the registered nurse in the insertion of external jugular peripherally inserted central lines (EJ PICC) and external jugular peripheral intravenous catheters (EJ PIV)*. Retrieved from www.ins1.org/files/public/08_26_08_INS_Position_Paper.pdf

Infusion Nurses Society. (2011). Infusion nursing standards of practice. *Journal of Infusion Nursing, 34*(1S). Retrieved from www.vardhandboken.se/Dokument/INS_2011.pdf

Ingles, L., Law, F., & Revell, A. (2010). The radiology nurse. *Inside Radiology*. Retrieved from www.insideradiology.com.au/pages/view.php?T_id=94

International Marketing Ventures. (2012). *2012 CT market outlook report* (pp. 7–45). Des Plaines, IL: International Marketing Ventures.

Jan, S., & Nardi, D. (2005). Radiology nursing and the Asian population. *Journal of Radiology Nursing, 24*(4), 79–84.

Jauch, E., Saver, J., Adams, J., Bruno, A., Connors, J., Damaerschalk, B., . . . Yonas, H. (2013). Guidelines for the early management of patients with acute ischemic stroke. *Stroke, 44*, 870–947. doi: 10.1161/STR.0b013e318284056a

Joint Commission Center for Transforming Healthcare. (2013, May 13). *Improving transitions of care: Handoff communication.* Retrieved from www.centerfortransforminghealthcare.org

Joint Commission International. (2007). *Joint Commission International accreditation standards for hospitals* (3rd ed.). Retrieved from www.jointcommission.org

Kalinowski, M., & Wagner, H. (2005). Sedation and pain management in interventional radiology. *C2I2, 111*(2). Retrieved from www.c2ic.deigithalamus.com/voll_iii_issue2

Kanal, E., Barkovich, A. J., Bell, C., Borgstede, J. P., Bradley, W. G., Froelich, J. W., . . . Hernandez, D. (2013). ACR guidance document on MR safe practices: 2013. *Journal of Magnetic Resonance Imaging, 37*, 501–530. doi:10.1002/jmri.24011

Kim, S., Lee, J., Lee, M., Kim, G., Han, J., & Choi, B. (2008). Sonography transmission gel as endorectal contrast agent for tumor visualization in rectal cancer. *American Journal of Roentgenology, 191*(1), 186–189.

Lee, C. H., Dershaw, D. D., Kopans, D., Evans, P., Monsees, B., Monticciolo, D., . . . Burhenne, L. W. (2010). Breast cancer screening with imaging: Recommendations from the Society of Breast Imaging and the ACR on the use of mammography, breast MRI, breast ultrasound, and other technologies for the detection of clinically occult breast cancer. *Journal of the American College of Radiology, 7*, 18–27.

Linder, J., & Schiska, A. (2007). Imaging children: Tips and tricks. *Journal of Radiology Nursing, 26*(1), 23–25.

Matich, S. (2011). Just pediatrics: Radiation and the pediatric patient. *Journal of Radiology Nursing, 30*(4), 170–171.

MedConditions. (2013). *Dictionary of medical conditions terminology.* Retrieved from medconditions.net

Meyers, J. L., & Chaudhuri, S. (2011). Procedural sedation and analgesia: A practical review for non-anesthesiologists. *Journal of Surgical Radiology, 2*(4), 344–356

Monsein, L. H., Jeffrey, P. J., van Heerden, B. B., Szabo, Z., Schwartz, J. R., Camargo, E. E., & Chazaly, J. (1991). Assessing adequacy of collateral circulation during balloon test occlusion of the internal carotid artery with 99m Tc-HMPAO SPECT. *AJNR. American Journal of Neuroradiology, 12*, 1045–1051.

Moody, E. B., Dawson, R. C., III, & Sandler, M. P. (1991). 99m Tc-HMPAO SPECT imaging in interventional neuroradiology: Validation of balloon test occlusion. *AJNR. American Journal of Neuroradiology, 12*, 1043–1044.

Munn, Z., & Jordan, Z. (2013). Interventions to reduce anxiety, distress, and the need for sedation in pediatric patients undergoing magnetic resonance imaging: A systematic review. *Journal of Radiology Nursing, 32*(2), 97–96.

Myers, T., Bolmers, M., Gregoric, I., Kar, B., & Frazier, H. (2009). Assessment of arterial blood pressure during support with an axial flow left ventricular assist device. *The Journal of Heart and Lung Transplantation, 28*(5), 423–427. doi:10.1016/j.healun.2009.01.013

National Institute on Alcohol Abuse and Alcoholism. (2013). *Alcohol use disorders.* Retrieved from www.niaaa.nih.gov/alcohol-health/overview-alcohol-consumption/alcohol-use-disorders

National Kidney Foundation. (2001). III. NKF-K/DOQI clinical practice guidelines for vascular access: Update 2000. *American Journal of Kidney Disease, 37*, S137–S181.

Occupational Safety and Health Administration. (n.d.). *Ionizing radiation.* Retrieved from www.osha.gov/SLTC/radiationionizing

Organisation for Economic Co-operation and Development. (2012). Magnetic resonance imaging (MRI) exams, total. *Health: Key Tables from OECD, 46.* doi:10.1787/mri-exam-total-table-2012-2-en

Ott, L., Pinsky, M., Hoffman, L., Clarke, S., Clark, S., Ren, D., & Hravnak, M. (2012). Medical emergency team calls in the radiology department: Patient characteristics and outcomes. *BMJ Quality and Safety, 21*(6), 509–518. doi:10.1136/bmjqs-2011-000423

Patel, I., Davidson, J., Nikolic, B., Salazar, G., Schwartzberg, M., Walker, T., & Saad, W. (2012). Consensus guidelines for periprocedural management of coagulation status and hemostasis risk in percutaneous image-guided interventions. *Journal of Vascular & Interventional Radiology, 23*(6), 727–736.

Peterman, S. B., Taylor, A., Jr., & Hoffman, J. C., Jr. (1991). Improved detection of cerebral hypoperfusion with internal carotid balloon test occlusion and Tc-HMPAO cerebral perfusion SPECT imaging. *AJNR. American Journal of Neuroradiology, 12,* 1035–1041.

Reilly, L., Byrne, A., & Ely, E. (2012). Does the use of an immobilizer provide a quality MR image of the brain in infants? *Journal of Radiology Nursing, 31*(3), 91–96.

Robbins, J., & Pozniak, M. (2010). *Contrast media tutorial.* Madison, WI: University of Wisconsin, Department of Radiology.

Roche, M., Diers, D., Duffield, C., & Catling-Paull, C. (2010). Violence toward nurses, the work environment, and patient outcomes. *Journal of Nursing Scholarship, 42*(1), 13–22.

Scovell, S. (2013, September 26). Laser and light therapy of lower extremity telangiectasias, reticular veins and small varicose veins. *Uptodate.com.*

Society of Nuclear Medicine and Molecular Imaging. (2013). *Practice guidelines.* Retrieved from interactive.snm.org/index.cfm?PageID=772

Sousa, M. (2013). Management and leadership: An agile approach to new nurse orientation: How one hospital created a sustainable orientation plan for newly hired radiology nurses. *Journal of Radiology Nursing, 32*(1), 45–47.

Spry, C. (1997). *Essentials of perioperative nursing.* Gaithersburg, MD: Aspen.

The Joint Commission. (2013). *Specifications manual for National Hospital Inpatient Quality Measures.* Retrieved from www.joint Thecommission.org

Tsushima, Y., Taketomi-Takahashi, A., Takei, H., Otake, H., & Endo, K. (2010). Radiation exposure from CT examinations in Japan. *BMC Medical Imaging, 10,* 24. Retrieved from www.biomedcentral.com/1471-2342/10/24

U.S. Food and Drug Administration. (2013). *Radiation-emitting products: Medical imaging.* Retrieved from www.fda.gov/Radiation-EmittingProducts/RadiationEmittingProductsandProcedures/MedicalImaging/default.htm

Vallerand, A. H., & Sanoski, C. A. (2012). *Davis's drug guide for nurses* (13th ed.). Philadelphia, PA: F. A. Davis.

Venkatesan, A. M., Kundu, S., Sacks, D., Wallace, M. J., Wojak, J. C., Rose, S. C., . . . Cardella, J. F. (2010). Practice guideline for adult antibiotic prophylaxis during vascular and interventional radiology procedures. *Journal of Vascular Interventional Radiology, 21*, 1611–1630.

Vidacare. (2013). *Intraosseous vascular access bibliography*. Retrieved from www.vidacare.com/files/EZ-IO_Articles-updated-080513.pdf

Waldman, D. (2013). *Ultrasound clinics interventional ultrasound* (Vol. 8, No. 2). Philadelphia, PA: Elsevier.

Warren, J., Fromm, R., Orr, R., Rotello, L., Horst, M., & American College of Critical Care Medicine. (2004). Guidelines for the inter- and intrahospital transport of critically ill patients. *Critical Care Medicine, 32*(1), 256–262.

Waszynski, C. M. (2007). Detecting delirium. *American Journal of Nursing, 107*(12), 50–59.

World Health Organization. (2007). *Communication during patient handovers, 1*(3). Retrieved from www.jointcommission international.org

Zimmermann, P. G. (2010). Revisiting IM injections. *American Journal of Nursing, 110*(2), 60–61.

Zimmermann, P. G. (2013). Workplace violence and disruptive behavior. In B. B. Hammond & P. G. Zimmermann (Eds.), *Sheehy's ENA manual of emergency care* (7th ed.). St. Louis, MO: Elsevier.

# Index